WHY DIDN'T SOMEBODY
TELL ME I WAS FAT?

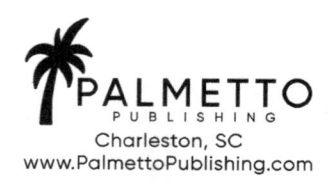

PALMETTO
PUBLISHING
Charleston, SC
www.PalmettoPublishing.com

Why Didn't Somebody Tell Me I Was Fat?
Copyright © 2023 by Vincent L. Howard

First Edition

-Paperback ISBN: 979-8-8229-2096-5
eBook ISBN: 979-8-8229-2097-2

WHY DIDN'T SOMEBODY TELL ME I WAS FAT?

VINCENT L. HOWARD

CONTENTS

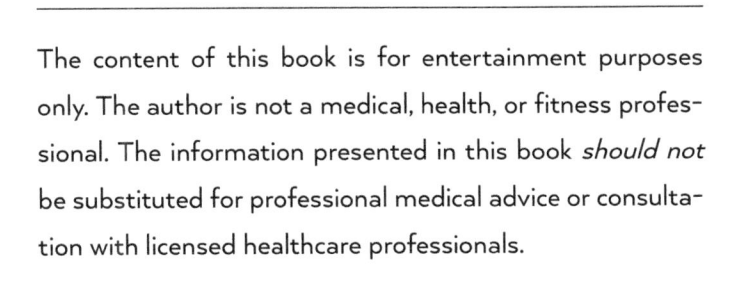

INTRODUCTION

IN ALL HONESTY, there is absolutely nothing wrong with being fat.

Seriously.

Because what is "fat" anyway? Who determines the weight or size at which people should feel good or bad? Does society get to decide? Fat is in the eye of the beholder, right?

Which is probably why nobody ever told me I was fat.

I was pretty fat, though. You know it's true too. Check the back cover again if you forgot.

It doesn't make me a bad person, but I was big. OK, OK—I was fat. Really fat. My point is that there's nothing wrong with it, and don't let anyone convince you otherwise. And even though not a single person ever said anything negative about my weight to my face, I have to admit I was getting a little tired of stopping to catch my breath going up the stairs, wearing the same clothes repeatedly because they were the only three things that fit, and sucking in my stomach when I was driving so I could safely turn the steering wheel.

I was tired of it, but I didn't know I was fat either. Kind of.

So I went on my merry way.

Eating.

I lost 120 or so pounds, eventually. I'm sharing my journey to let you know someone understands, and you can do it, too, if *you* want to. Fair warning, though: losing weight is like parenting or leading people. The basic principles are the same, but not everyone does it the same way. What worked for me may not work for you. I was kind of a nut you might not want to copy—we'll see in a little bit.

And don't forget the disclaimer. I'm not a doctor. I'm not a trainer or a fitness expert. Some of what I did is probably unhealthy. Some of what I did is *definitely* unhealthy. Just remember: I'm not telling you what to do. I'm telling you what I did in hopes of entertaining you for a few hours.

My hope is you'll see from my journey you can do it if you want to. And you might pick up a little encouragement to get to wherever it is you want to be. Or if you have extra-nutty tendencies, maybe you'll want to copy the healthy and good part of what I did, if any parts like that exist. But even if you disagree with everything I'm about to tell you, even if you read it and believe I'm a lunatic, a liar who's making up stories to try to be funny, or even if you think I'm a brilliant, innovative genius (it could happen), regardless of whatever else you get from my story, I hope you remember this:

There's nothing wrong with being fat.

Even so, somebody could've told me.

Let's get into my story.

CHAPTER 1

THAT'S WHERE THE HAPPY PEOPLE GO

THIS IS ACTUALLY a love story. It all began innocently enough, and because it was love, how could anyone possibly blame me? Because when love strikes, you're powerless to resist if you're human—and I'm human. Maybe it was hormones. It probably was. Those things are pretty powerful.

According to science, there are signs that tell you when you're in love, and looking back, it's clear my love was as real as it gets; it passed all the tests.

Thinking it's special. Oh, for sure. Special and magnificent. A one-of-a-kind love affair. Undoubtedly. They sing songs about the kind of love I felt. Old-school songs, at that.

Focusing on the positives. There were negatives, of course, like with any love affair. I didn't care. I was too blind to see anything but the positives, which outweighed the negatives.

Emotional instability. Unfortunate but true. I was so sad when we were apart for too long. Perhaps a mark of immaturity, but I was a teenager, so what do you expect?

Intensifying attraction. I was more in love every time we met. My love had no limit. I was out of control, but I liked the feeling. I loved the feeling, actually. It felt good. It felt right.

Intrusive thinking. Love was always on my mind. I couldn't stop thinking about love. I didn't *want* to stop thinking about love. It was the kind of love that makes you write names and draw pictures in your notebooks. Yes, boys do that too.

Emotional dependency. When it was good, I was complete. When it was bad, I couldn't quite function properly. I needed my love in a way I had never needed anything before.

Planning a future. What can we do tomorrow? Next week? Next month? We will always be together, right? Good—because I cannot imagine a future without my love.

Yes. It was love that did it. My first love. Love at first sight. And you never forget your first love, do you?

For me—it was pancakes.

That's not a nickname (thankfully).

I mean, it was pancakes. Real ones. As in the kind made with flour and eggs.

It was my mama who introduced me to my beloved pancakes. I wasn't aware of it at the time, but pancakes are really cheap to make. Flour or Bisquick, couple of eggs, add water—that's all it takes. Back then, if she was in a good mood, my mom would slap it all together and we'd have pancake eating contests on Saturday mornings. You would think after six pancakes...eight pancakes...ten pancakes... someone would get tired of pancakes. Never happened. Not once, so...Mama kept 'em comin'. This was the 1970s, so it was a long time ago, but I'm fairly sure our family record was sixteen pancakes. And the usual winner was...who cares? Everyone got to win. It was *pancakes*, remember?

All good things come to an end eventually, so when doughnuts came on the scene later, I didn't see pancakes as much. I mean, it's not like you can carry pancakes with you while walking around, right?

You can't drive with pancakes in the passenger seat, keeping syrup and butter in the glove compartment, right? A nice dream, maybe, but it's not safe.

Nobody could blame me for switching; I'd found a new love. Maybe I'd still be in love with pancakes if someone came up with a drive-through pancake restaurant. Wait, McDonald's has those now, don't they? Oh well…it came too late; I had already moved on. Still, I never, ever stopped loving my precious pancakes.

Pancakes and doughnuts may have been my early favorites, but I've been in love with food all my life. The food names changed, but I kept on loving whatever food was in front of me with sincerity and intensity. I guess that makes me kind of a food playboy, doesn't it? In hindsight, that also would have been a great name for this book.

Or maybe I developed into a "compulsive eater." I didn't Google that—I got that term from an episode of *Three's Company*. You probably don't remember that episode when Jack and Chrissy had a bet about whether Chrissy could give up food longer than Jack could give up women. And Jack tricked Chrissy into eating chocolate cake, so she lost. Funny episode. I think '70s television is where we got fast information before Googling was a thing.

I wonder why I remember that episode, though. You already know: food playboy or compulsive eater…it's kind of the same thing. If it has to do with food, I'll probably remember.

I was telling my mom the other day how, even though we were poor, I don't remember ever being truly hungry while growing up. She got indignant when she claimed we weren't poor; I had to remind her, "Mom, we lived in the mountains in the car. A few years later, we made our Christmas presents by hand and wrapped them in newspaper."

Then Mama was like, "Oh yeah—well, in that case, I did a good job of keeping my babies husky and fed, huh?"

Yes, she absolutely did. Love you, Mama! Shout out to Miss Rose; that's what you can call my mama. If 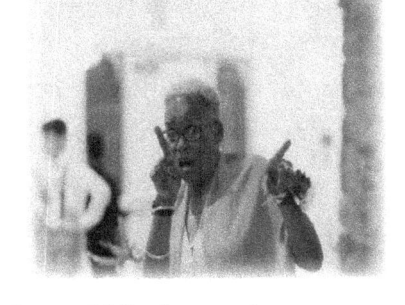 you were writing a book, you'd find a random way to include *your* mama too.

Even though I don't ever remember being hungry, food has always been a treat for me and my brothers. I remember when my parents would have their friends over when I was a child. Back in those days, when the grown folks came over to drink and play cards, kids stayed in their own rooms and out of sight. In addition to entertaining ourselves in our room back then, we planned missions—not to free prisoners or anything like that, of course, but to recover snacks. That made us like Rambo before Rambo was Rambo. Or even better—we were like the Borg in *Star Trek*, feeling like "resistance is futile." Get it? As in, "Don't try to keep us from the deliciousness"? Wait, you're not a Trekkie? *Star Trek: The Next Generation* wasn't even out then anyway. No problem—I'm sure you get the picture.

We'd send my baby brother out as a distraction while my other little brother snuck in to snatch up the chips, pretzels, little sandwiches, cold pizza slices, or whatever else they had out there. Then we'd bring it back to our room for my older brother and me to split it all up among the four of us boys.

Then again, sometimes we'd just wait for the adults to get drunk. That was a somewhat foolproof strategy too. Actually better. Because it was quicker.

Later on, I'd be on my way to Bell Junior High, and I'd stop at my friend Robbie's house. I told my mom we needed to study together or check homework before school, but Robbie's mom usually went to work early. That made it a perfect opportunity to whip up some pancakes before school. It was a thirty-minute walk to Bell, so it only made sense to have a pancake snack to keep our strength up during the long walk. It *did* keep our strength up, too, along with the knowledge that school breakfast was waiting for us once we got there. I'm not sure if schools provide breakfast anymore. If not, that's a pity. Good times—they served pancakes too.

It wasn't just pancakes, though. I told you, for us food playboys, if the pancakes weren't there, we'd fall in love with whatever food happened to be there; that's what playboys do. Like for birthdays: our birthday celebrations usually consisted of being "king of the house" for the day, when everyone except Mama had to do whatever we said, and you got to pick whatever you wanted to eat. I wonder what it says when a kid gets to pick whatever he wants for his birthday dinner and exclaims he wants hot dogs *with* chili? I should have asked for more than meat that boils on the stove for fifteen minutes covered with canned beans, but what did I know? Seemed like a delicious idea at the time.

Then there'd be times we'd take the Greyhound bus to Texas to visit my grandparents. Those were exciting trips. I'd always sit with one of my younger brothers, and without fail, we'd wake up before the sun came up and be the only ones awake, letting the adults

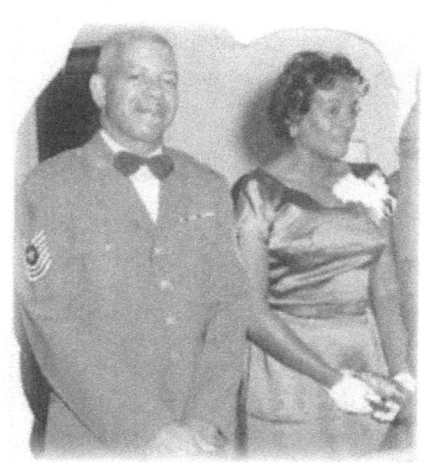

snore while we whispered and giggled as the bus hurtled through the darkness. We had a child's excitement about where the bus was going to stop for breakfast when the sun came up and what we were going to eat when we got there.

Then, when we got to Texas, my grandparents took us to church every Sunday. And let me be clear:

Every. Single. Sunday. The African Methodist Episcopalian denomination stayed in church for eighty dozen hours too. *However*, no matter how long church lasted, it was all about Furr's Cafeteria after church on Sundays. I loved that buffet. It was "all you can eat."

Later, I started playing Little League baseball. I think our uniforms were yellow and white. I don't remember our team's name or who coached it; I don't remember how many games we won, but I think it was none. I don't remember a single person who was on my team. I sure do remember those cheeseburger baskets we got after the games, though; those were the best cheeseburgers and fries of all time. Plus, there was a place called Mama Jo's around the corner with the thickest, greasiest, cheesiest pepperoni pizza on earth. I couldn't wait for the games to end so I could dig in.

You can find more detailed stories about cheeseburger baskets and pizza in my book *Crossroads: The Long Way Home*—available on Amazon now.

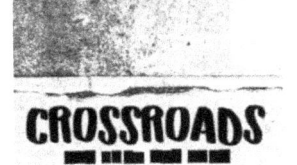

OK, that was a shameless plug. I apologize. Is that even allowed? I can violate my own copyright, can't I? I was kind of kidding anyway. I probably won't do it again. Let's get back to the food.

Let me introduce you to my father. My Pops was the real deal; life got much better after Pops came on the scene to take care of us, make the tasty greens, barbecue, provide that Southern wisdom, and come to my track meets to cheer, even when I lost. My Pops was smart; plus, he'd been in the Army during the 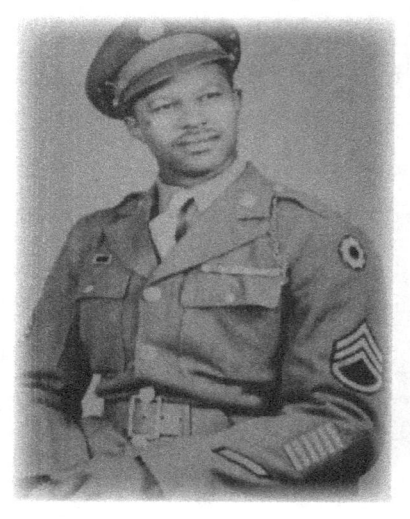 war. He knew ambush missions when he saw them. He knew his boys went on food recon patrol every night because we were true food predators—night stalkers who would attack the kitchen as soon as we heard Pops's cowboy movies turn off and the lights click off for the evening. We were an enemy force, intent on nightly missions to ambush and overwhelm Pops's food budget.

So Pops put a lock on the food pantry.

That's a strong move, but he had to do it. Does that sound harsh? Maybe. But the problem was if he hadn't locked up the pantry, a month's worth of food wouldn't have even survived one week. Ever the brilliant tactician, Pops found an old-school method of locking food up at night.

It worked for a night or two until my brothers and I found a *new*-school method of picking the lock.

And once we figured that out, we were pirates who had found the buried treasure; except our treasure was peanut butter...cookies...peanut butter cookies...Twinkies...Ding Dongs...Pop-Tarts...and our favorite, the cereal. Oh, the colors and the boxes they came in were truly *beautiful*! Frosted Flakes, Trix, Cocoa Puffs, Fruity Pebbles, Razor Blades—that's what we called Cap'n Crunch. If you ever ate any, I know you understand.

This wasn't as easy as it may sound. First you had to go in the kitchen without making any noise, and you couldn't turn on the lights, because that would blow your cover. You had to pick the pantry lock in the dark, get the food, eat the food, clean up any dishes, clean and dry the sink, take any trash with you to the bathroom to flush it, put the food back in the pantry, and relock the pantry. *Then* there was the part about getting back into bed before Pops woke up and came to investigate. We figured nine-minute stealth missions were safe. In and out.

As my food playboy life continued, I arrived at prom night right before graduation. Do you know where my prom was? Me neither. Who did I go with? Good question; I forgot. Some dark-haired girl. I think her name was Jackie…or Stephanie…or something else. Or was it Kelly? I've always thought it was something that ended in that "e" sound. Whatever.

I do remember two things with crystal clarity, though. One, I wore a baby-blue tux with ruffles and tails, which is significant, because these kids today don't get clean like we got clean back in the day—I was *sharp*. And two, I remember we went to Benihana's for the pre-prom dinner, and I was absolutely amazed at the chef doing all that slicing, dicing, and flipping with the knives and food. As far as I was concerned, it was the greatest show on Earth. OK, so I have low standards and am easily impressed. Sue me.

I made it through high school and headed off to college at West Texas State University in Canyon, Texas. I've been honest with you guys up to this point, so let me be real with you: I have no idea how I graduated high school, much less got into college. I had to take a biology test that last week of high school, or I wouldn't have graduated. I can't believe I passed that final test either. I was just picking answers at random to get it over with, so clearly my school didn't want to see me anymore.

I don't remember filling out any admissions applications, applying for financial aid, or anything like that. I don't even remember registering for any classes. Somehow, I got registered as an accounting major. However it happened, I was there—West Texas State University!

Except I didn't feel like going to any classes. I hated school back then.

I hate saying I hated school; what kind of message is that for the children?

But I hated school.

I guess I don't hate saying it as much as I thought I did.

I went to my classes a couple of times, then stopped going. I couldn't help it; college classes made me sleepy. All of them. I wasn't sure what to do with myself after I decided I wasn't going to any more classes. What does a seventeen-year-old do when they're enrolled in college, over a thousand miles away from home for the first time, but they're not going to any classes?

Well—they flunk out of school.

Didn't pass a single class. Straight Fs: 0.00 grade point average. Lowest grades in the history of recorded academics. My spectacular failure allowed my seventeen-year-old mind to formulate a philosophy that sustained me back then and provided a purpose. A path. A vision. Goals. A new life doctrine that would sustain me for decades was born during those days:

"When in doubt…eat."

There were a bunch of cafeterias on the campus, and since I had a student ID, I didn't need money; come on in, and just like Furr's cafeteria, it was "all you can eat," buffet style. My favorite dining facility was the one close by Jarrett Hall, the athletic dorm. It had big glass windows and was so huge, you could see the buffet table from the street. I even got a job there as a dishwasher. I would sneak off to grab some deliciousness off the buffet table when I was supposed to be going to the bathroom. I did about thirteen bathroom breaks every four-hour shift.

My big brother was a student there too. One day, he pulled me to the side like any good big brother should do and told me, "You have to study and work hard, Vincent. You're not in high school anymore; this is college. No one is giving away free grades. You have to go to class *sometimes*. Do you want to study together?"

My brother. A good man. Skinny too. He's a professor at Baylor University today. I considered his offer.

Didn't line up in any way with my new philosophy, though. So I told him, "Sorry, big bro. No can do."

Obviously, college was a bust. Soon after I left, I was on my own, and I had to enter the world of work—but work was hard to come by.

I lied. It wasn't too hard to come by, but work got in the way of everything that was fun, so I didn't chase work that hard. I stumbled into a blood bank by chance—they offered $6, juice, and a doughnut for a pint of blood. Now consider: the minimum wage then was $2.50 an hour, so for some blood that I had a body full of, I got two-plus hours of salary *and* food?

Sold.

I found out where all the blood banks in the city were and considered it my new job. Give blood, sip sone juice, eat a doughnut, then take the bus or walk to the next blood bank. Put it all together, and I had a few bucks for a daily burrito, some rolled tacos, and maybe a cinnamon roll.

That gig worked for me. Until I found the military, that is.

People normally join the military for a variety of reasons: patriotism, college benefits, training for the future, travel, and many other noble reasons.

I joined because my friend bought me two McDonald's value meals on the same day.

Brian came home on leave from the Marine Corps, and I can't front; I was tired, dirty, and funky, because the blood banks had started measuring my internal levels of something, and whatever they were measuring, mine was too low or too high, so they stopped letting me give blood.

I think they call that getting laid off.

As we sat in McDonald's, by the time Brian had bought me that second value meal, I knew this military thing was worth checking out. I mean, a value meal is one thing, but *two* value meals? Clearly, my friend was living *large*. Plus that purple gear he had on was cold.

I went to the recruiter's office soon after. He said a lot, but I was dreaming about the chow halls he told me about. I never admit that when I'm speaking to groups now. This is the first time I've disclosed my sustenance obsessions, but I was really looking forward to those three squares a day. And why not? I was still in great shape.

I was a solid 180 pounds. Healthy and strong.

That's probably why my recruiter didn't tell me I was fat.

CHAPTER 2

GAMES PEOPLE PLAY

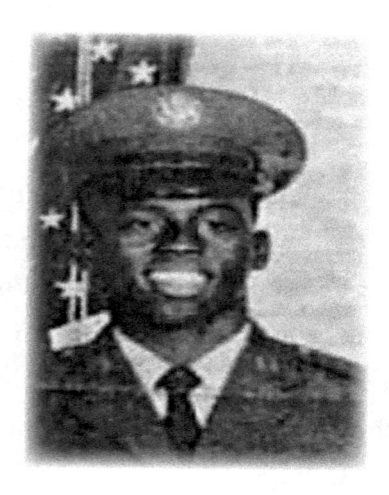

I GAINED TEN pounds by the time I graduated from basic training. I couldn't figure that out, though, at the time, I can't say I put a whole lot of effort into thinking about it. The thing was, I knew I had weighed 178 pounds in high school because I'd had to get on the scale for my high school football team. I'd gained two pounds over the next two years; I knew because I had to be weighed during my initial military physical, and I was 180 pounds. Six weeks later, I was all the way up to 190. Why?

In basic training, we were always on the go. Up before dawn, doing details, running everywhere, keeping active during the day, and exercising about every day, although football training was much tougher. Nevertheless, gaining ten pounds in six weeks is a very significant weight gain. I attribute it to two factors—for one thing, in basic training we had to eat fast. Really fast. Picture an empty table. One guy marches up and stands at attention holding a tray of food behind an empty chair. Then another person joins him, standing there in front of the table. Then a third person joins.

Finally, the last person comes, and when everyone is standing there, the last person commands, "Sit." And everyone sits. Then he says, "Pray," and you all bow your heads together, whether you're praying or not; I'm guessing some guys who never prayed before started praying in basic training.

Then he says, "Recover," and you lift your head up. Then he says, "Eat." And everyone starts eating. No talking. Just eating.

Because you only have ten minutes maximum to finish. Maybe less. If they catch you talking, the drill instructors assume you are finished, and they come over and end your meal prematurely. And I guess eating fast makes you more likely to eat more food than you need, which leads to weight gain. Now I have a confession: I Googled that little tidbit of information. It makes sense, though; eating fast doesn't seem healthy, does it? Now I know why. Only took me forty years to figure it out. Eating fast is bad. Got it.

Now here's the other thing. In basic training, there's no going back for second helpings. No time for all that. When you go through the food line, you'd better get what you want to eat, because if you don't, those hours to the next meal might as well be an eternity. So we piled the food on our plates. One problem, though: before you can leave, you have to show your plate to the drill instructor on duty. And if you didn't finish it all? Oh man, those DIs lose their minds! One time I saw them dump all the food on the floor and make every recruit at the table eat it; another time the DI took all the extra food on the guy's plate, divided it up among all four people at the table, and made everyone finish the food together. Unbelievable, right?

For good reason. I'm just kidding; they don't do that. It'd be hilarious if they did it to somebody else other than me, but all they do is scream or make you take a few extra bites. No big deal. I'll let you in on a secret that everyone knows: military retirees always stretch the truth a little. Sometimes we stretch it a lot. For example, I've been known to tell my children about battles I fought during Vietnam. I've told them I was the unsung hero in the Battle of the Wang Chung Valley but that my involvement was classified. It's very entertaining, but I don't know why we tell those stories. I'll stick to only absolute facts for the rest of the book. I promise.

Anyway, the thing is, I'm betting I had a few extra and unnecessary calories on my plate, and that was another factor leading to weight gain. Plus, people under stress eat differently. They're more likely to find comfort in food. And there was certainly a lot of stress in basic training. Like, the first night of basic training, the drill instructor screamed at all of us to *"Get in bed now!"* So I did—with all my clothes on. The instructor asked me if I was a f——idiot. I didn't answer; I just lay there feeling like one, but I was thinking, "But you said *now*."

Stress.

Then there were inspections. We had to fold everything in six-inch squares. Not five-and-a-half-inch squares, not five-and-seven-eighths-inch squares. Six-inch squares exactly. A lot of my flight mates snuck in a ruler that they passed around so everyone could measure their underwear. Me? Nah. I figured I could get it close enough. I failed many of those inspections. Sometimes I got yelled at, but sometimes everyone got punished if I messed up, even though they all did it right.

Stress.

And I got in a fight in basic training. Some kid called me a name that was an instant trigger—I bet you can guess the name too. Rhymes with "trigger."

Then, after he dropped that "trigger" bomb on me, he ran downstairs to get into formation, where he was supposedly safe, standing quietly at attention with the rest of the flight. He knew that in formation, with all the drill instructors around, nothing was going to happen. And I wasn't going to snitch; that went without saying. I was stuck, but everyone was looking at me to see what I was going to do. I could have gotten him later, I guess, but I couldn't let it pass with everyone staring at me like they were. When I rushed downstairs, I saw he was standing at attention in formation.

And he grinned at me.

So, drill instructors or no drill instructors, I dropped him. I had to. Wasn't much of a fight, though; it was more like I punched the guy…the guy fell down…fight was over. The stress occurred every day *after* the fight—because the drill instructors made me and Mr. Trigger Guy team up on just about everything after that.

It's easy to imagine how basic training was extra stressful on a variety of levels. As a stress reliever, I began looking forward to chow time, because even though that Mr. Trigger kid was somehow always at my table, the chow was good, and if you knew the rules, nobody screamed at you. Therefore, like many, I ate for comfort. Now I don't know about you, but when it comes to being comforted by food, I get a lot less comfort from a cold, hard apple than I get from some warm apple pie. I piled it on every day. No vegetables or healthy food, though—comfort food only.

Put it all together, and I gained ten pounds in six short weeks. Ever see that commercial with that one lady dancing around like an idiot, being "super-pumped" about gaining sixty-five pounds? Well—if that's what you want, no need to buy whatever she's selling. I'm giving away the secret free of charge: eat fast, eat bad, and always clean your plate, no matter what you put on it, and you can be "super-pumped" too. Hopefully, you feel the sarcasm dripping from that statement.

I eventually completed training as an Air Force medic, and my first permanent duty station was Offutt Air Force Base, Nebraska. And who do you think my roommate was? Or more importantly, what do you think his job was? He was a military chef, which is another way of saying he worked in the 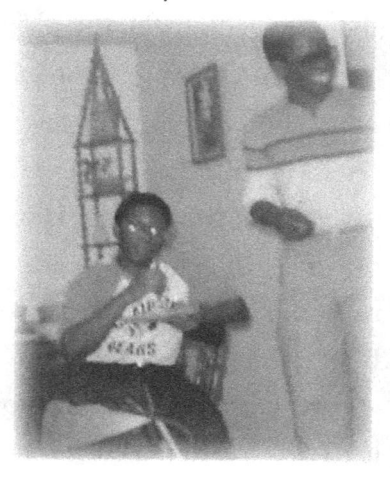 chow hall, but he was a talented cook. Even to this day, he puts recipes out on social media, and if you knew what I know, you'd be putting this book down to Google his recipes or look him up. So it's just as well.

We weren't allowed food in the barracks, but I had the "master chef" in my room, who sometimes brought unauthorized food home, plus we had a chow hall on the first floor of the barracks. Not every barracks had a chow hall, but ours did. And that meant our nostrils got caressed by the smell of bacon frying for 150 airmen every single day. And just like with my childhood pancake eating contests, did I get tired of it? Not a chance. I wonder if smelling food makes you more likely to want to eat more? I'm not going to cheat this time; no running off to Google to make myself look like I know what I'm talking about. When you get a chance, go take a look for yourself—I bet smells trigger hunger hormones that make us want to eat. Just a guess. I bet I'm right, though.

I worked in the hospital, which was about five miles away from the barracks, so the hospital had a chow hall too. I was surrounded by food everywhere, but I wasn't exactly mad about that. We were surrounded by food all day and even at night; since military operations are conducted around the clock, the airmen who were working swing shift and during the midnight hours had to eat too, right? That's why the Air Force had what we called "midnight chow."

The chow hall would open from 10:00 p.m. to 1:00 a.m. to feed personnel who were working at night. Anyone could go though. The only rules were that you had to be in uniform and you couldn't take any food to go. You had to eat it there in the chow hall. So what did we do? We went, of course! We'd go to the Airmen's Club to drink, come back to the barracks to change into our uniforms, go grab a cheese omelet and some French toast, stumble back to the barracks, change clothes again, and head back to the Airmen's Club.

You might ask, "All that for some eggs?"

Answer: "Yes. It was all for the eggs. With cheese. And bread with syrup on it."

Sometimes we'd go even if we hadn't been to the club; someone would bang on the door, and you knew we were getting ready to make a midnight chow run. I think there's something about eating at midnight. Google that, too, when you get a chance. I bet it's a thing. Could also be that we needed to get out of our rooms. With three men to a room, it was tight in there, and it was good to just get out every chance we got.

Next up was an assignment to Montana and the most brutal, nose-hair-freezing, block-heater-using cold I'd ever felt—which came with a whole new set of issues. Montana is a place where, if you like to hunt, fish, or do things in the snow, you are going to absolutely love being stationed there. Unfortunately for me, I'm a city guy from San Diego. I don't fish, I don't do snow stuff, and the only hunting I like to do is hunting for peanut butter and jelly in the middle of the night. So what is there to do during off time for a guy like me? Just guess.

Drink alcohol.

Yes—and eat too.

I know, and you know, and I know you know that drinking lowers inhibitions and reduces discipline to about zero. We'd drink, eat, go to work, come home and drink, eat some more, and so on and so on. Montana had a bunch of food options like elk and bison too. I guess that's healthy, but I took a pass. I never tried it, not one time. Besides, even if I wanted it, I'd have had to go get it, and it was cold out there.

Our preference was having food delivered to us and letting the Montana natives deal with all that snow and those icy roads. You know what that meant? It meant we lived on pizza. For three years.

And alcohol. And playing my favorite *Super Mario Brothers* video game until deep into the early morning. And eating more pizza. Not proud of it, but you need to know how I got to where I got, right?

I did get a temporary respite, though: I found martial arts. American Kenpō, to be exact. Now I have nothing but respect for martial arts philosophies and the history behind them and the katas and the colored belts and all that. If pressed, I might even remember a technique or two, and if you catch me in the right moment, you might even convince me to demonstrate my favorite martial arts strike and the only one I happen to remember—my oh-so-deadly chicken kick.

With all due respect to my chicken kick, the techniques, and the Zen and mystical mystics, I just wanted to spar. I'd boxed in college, and I've always loved boxing. Having to spar made me eat right, or at least better. I was still a food playboy, but I was occasionally cheating on my fatty foods with vegetables and fish. As in tuna fish sandwiches. I've never admitted that before. Feels good to come clean.

I was sparring against black belts, full contact, so my sensei didn't bother putting me in forms competitions to see who had the best kata. I wanted to fight, I was good at it, and he knew it. Sensei entered me into the open heavyweight division. I felt strong too. And I felt ready until I got into the locker room and asked around about who I was fighting. When I saw him warming up, I thought, "Whew, he looks *more* ready."

Once I got in the ring, I saw the crowd filling up. I was the last fight before the professional kickboxers started, so the crowd had started to drink and get rowdy. I wished I'd been down in the crowd drinking with them, or that I had at least been less of a cheating food playboy. Too late, though; it was time to fight.

I started the fight out well; I wasn't scared anymore—a fight's a fight, right? Then, that guy kicked me in the face so hard, I thought I was dreaming. I didn't know if I was awake or asleep, lying on my back or standing on my knees; I was what they call "out on my feet." I could hear, though; the crowd was screaming for that guy to kill me. And he would have if he had attacked. He told me later he didn't realize I was hurt so badly. That's a nice skill to have; the opponent doesn't always have to know you've been hurt. That's true in life too.

Since he didn't attack, once my vision and the feeling in my legs returned, I attacked. And I didn't make the mistake he made; when I got him hurt, I poured it on, and the referee stopped the fight in the first round. I was happy to get out of there. I was 208 pounds for this fight, and I was looking forward to doing it again, but the military reassigned me.

Next stop was overseas. Looking back, it was the first time in several years my recreational focus did not involve food and alcohol. Well—it still kind of involved alcohol, but I had to get in shape again, because my base had a tackle football team, and I intended to try out. All the marine bases had teams too; there were ten total teams in the area. I made the team; in fact, I made the Pacific Stars & Stripes sports section. For this game against Camp Kinser, I ran for 180 yards and two touchdowns. That's sig-nificant for two reasons: (1) I've been waiting three

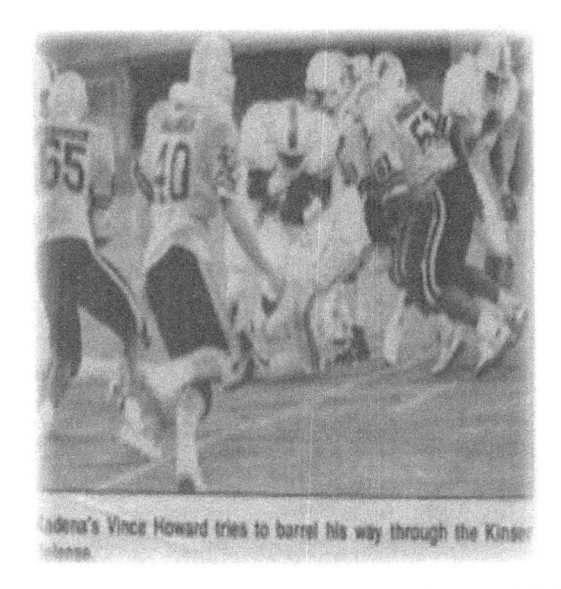

adena's Vince Howard tries to barrel his way through the Kinser

decades to talk about that game and post this Stars & Stripes picture *somewhere*, and (2) I know my weight had climbed to 218 pounds; I know because I remember weighing myself because of football. Listen, though; I was an athletic 218—muscular, powerful, fast, like you might expect from a star running back, which I humbly submit I was back then. I was quite the specimen during those days.

Who would have guessed at the time that physically, it was all downhill from there?

That was the last year they played tackle football overseas. Something about the budget or some other probably good reason I didn't care about, like there were too many people getting injured. For me, it was back to eating and drinking for the next three years. I needed sports or something positive to do with my time. Not that food isn't a positive thing—clearly it is—but remember my philosophy?

When in doubt…eat.

I had a chance to fight again against a marine named Royce Hussman. I kind of got in shape. Let me stop lying; I was in horrible fight shape. I never stopped my playboy eating; I never stopped drinking; I never stopped smoking cigarettes; I just did a lot of working out. It showed the night I fought in a downtown arena too; I was exhausted after thirty seconds of fighting. Asian crowds are quiet when watching sports, so I had to be extra careful. Every time Royce punched me in the face, which was about five hundred times or so, I wanted to yell, "Ouch!" or "Hey, that hurts!" or "Knock it off!"—but I thought the loud echo of my screams would be a little embarrassing.

Royce slapped me around for the entire three rounds. He didn't hit that hard, but his hands were so fast, and his technique was amazing. He would make this move with his footwork, and I would glance down at what he had just done. It was like I forgot I was in a fight, but unfortunately for me, Royce didn't forget. If I made the miscalculation of glancing down to admire his footwork, even for a second, my reward was another punch in the face. Sometimes two or three.

And unlike me, he was not getting tired. He was smiling while I felt the weight of every double cheeseburger I'd eaten while I was supposed to be training. I knew I was going to lose this fight, but toward the end of the third round, I threw a lazy, sloppy punch that landed with pure luck; Royce fell, and he didn't get up.

I'd never been so exhausted in my life.

I was 228 pounds for that fight; I was approaching thirty years old, and I'd picked up thirty-eight extra pounds over the past decade. Four pounds a year doesn't seem like a lot, but it is.

For the first time, I was having to buy shirts in a larger size. I even had to buy a couple of XXL-sized shirts, depending on the cut.

But even so, at least, nobody told me I was fat.

CHAPTER 3

ONCE YOU GET STARTED

WITH MY OVERSEAS tour of duty now complete, it was time for me to head back stateside—to Utah, specifically. For a while there, it was straight-up party time, because I didn't have a car, and I was back to living in the barracks. Why? It's a long story. Well, it's not that long or even that complicated, but it doesn't fit with the topic of this book. It's an interesting tale, though; I promise to tell it to you in detail in my next book.

When I wasn't working, I was mostly hanging out at the NCO Club on Hill Air Force Base. Understand this, though: I'm definitely not a "club guy." I saw the club life similar to the way I see social media today; I didn't understand the rules, I found it difficult to be myself, and I doubted the pictures ev-

eryone was painting of themselves. I saw personas—
people in the club who I knew did not really act the
way they portrayed themselves in the club. I see the
same thing on social media.

Just like with the social media scene today, I nav-
igated the club scene back then because that's how

people were "social."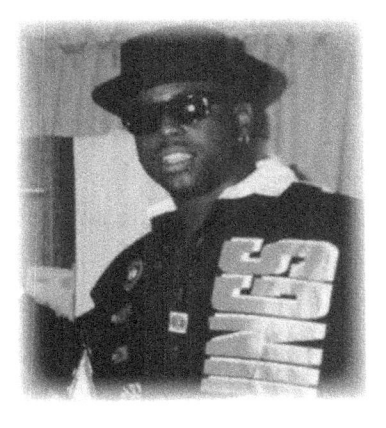
Bottom line, though,
I found the club scene
phony, and it was just
way too crowded for me.
Many find it difficult to
believe I'm a hard-core
introvert by nature. I'm
not shy; that's some-
thing different. I'm not even the quiet type. Still, I'm
also not the type to hang out in the club. Don't let my
cool hat fool ya.

Even when I was younger, I found it boring, because it was the same thing happening over and over.
And it's too loud. And I got sleepy. I guess I was old
before I really got old. Either that or maybe I'm just
more of a "dominoes and spades," kick-it-at-the-
crib kind of guy, but hey, I was in Utah. It's not like

there was a whole lot to do; remember what I told you about Montana? Well, this was kind of the same thing. Without the elk.

So it was to the club I went, three or four times a week. I probably should have taken some college classes or done something else positive, but there I was, feeling the boredom set in, night after night, over and over. My answer to the boredom: I drank more alcohol to make it fun. I was not just an introvert, but I was also a square—a square with cool '90s clothes, but still a square. I got more of a kick out of watching the people with constant drinks in my hand; that's what I did as opposed to going with the normal club flow. Watching the people was interesting. I'd watch someone, and it'd be funny to watch them get drunker and drunker, going from person to person, dancing by themselves but pretending to be dancing on the floor in the crowd like they were having a ball.

Wait. I was drinking too. Was I drunk? That might have been *me* I saw. I forgot. Well, whoever it was, I definitely remember those were some fuzzy, crazy days.

Then, thankfully, when the lights came on and everyone was leaving, it was finally time to go home, right?

No.

Time to go to Denny's.

At a minimum, that's drinking massive amounts of liquor about four times a week. Then, if there was no work the next day, and sometimes even if there *was* work the next day, add an order of Moons over My Hammy or an Ultimate Slam. The pancakes remained forever delicious, but after that, it was heading straight to bed with all those calories sitting in my gut. Then I'd always *want* to get up and work out, but the older I got and the more rank I earned, the easier it got to say, "Bleh—next time" or "I'm too busy." Even if I made a plan to work out in the evening, it didn't always pan out, because I'd gone out drinking the night before; either I was exhausted and needed to catch up on rest, or I was headed out again and needed to rest up for later festivities.

I was still working out, though. I was hoping to get more chances to fight in between going to the club several times a week and the late-night dominoes-and-spades sessions that involved a snack fest, along with the liquor that never stopped flowing. Even though I was getting some workouts in, I could tell I wasn't getting the same bang out of my gym sessions. My clothes kept getting tighter, for one thing. In my mind, I figured they were probably shrinking in the dryer. Or maybe they used different, cheaper materials in Utah to make clothes. And in the gym, I wasn't getting stronger. I was lifting and working out as hard as I ever had, but I was getting *weaker*. I couldn't push the same weight I was used to pushing, and I couldn't figure it out. Perhaps it was because my workouts were getting more and more sporadic? Or worse: surely I wasn't getting old?

Well, maybe a little, but there was more to it than that.

The alcohol had something to do with it too.

Alcohol was softening me up. I know I was heavier; I could feel it. But I was still looking and feeling good, so my mind was constantly playing tricks on me. I fooled myself, and it was all due to that boogie juice.

Since I'm no scientist, I'm gonna kind of paraphrase this next part. What I'm getting ready to say will not be exactly scientifically perfect, but I think

I have a good basic understanding of the issue, so here goes.

Alcohol has those empty calories; I know you know what that means. That's adding one thousand calories or more on club nights, and those calories don't do jack but make you want to take in even more food calories after the club closes. Alcohol also had me eating heavier the next morning to "soak up the alcohol." By the way—is that a thing? That's something we should Google: "soaking up the leftover alcohol" from last night doesn't exactly sound scientific, does it? I bet the club people out there know what I'm talking about. Fatty, unhealthy foods soak up all the alcohol in your system. I don't know why that is. It's one of those "club laws" that just seem to make sense.

Now I didn't know this then, but I found out later: excessive alcohol consumption increases glucose production in your body. Or at least in some bodies. Everyone processes alcohol differently, but clearly, I had one of those alcohol-glucose factory bodies. And glucose is sugar. So if your body is producing a bunch of sugar over time that it doesn't burn, what happens to the sugar?

I bet you know. No need for you this time, Google; we got this one.

Unburned sugar turns into fat.

And once my body got good at producing glucose, it kept right on doing it, whether I was drinking alcohol or not. So a type 2 diabetic was born.

But there's more.

I didn't know this at the time either, but I found out later that excessive alcohol consumption *also* increases estrogen production, even in men. Estrogen is a female hormone that women need for…I don't really know exactly, but I know it's a hormone women need. Men have estrogen, too, but not as much of it. I'm trying not to run to Google every other paragraph, because, for one thing, there was no Google back then, and I'm not trying to make myself seem smarter than I really was. We'll just keep with the basic knowledge that I knew was true even way back then.

Men don't want to be overflowing with estrogen; it makes it harder to build muscle. Similar to the glucose, once my body got used to producing it, my body just said, "OK, we must need it. Hormone system? Keep that estrogen coming, please." That's how alcohol made me soft. The truly annoying thing estrogen does when it comes to men is that estrogen makes it harder for the body to produce the male hormone testosterone.

And I love my testosterone. It's Man Stuff 101. I love my testosterone even more than pancakes. So, men, it's unfortunate that whether drinking alcohol or not drinking alcohol, our bodies start producing less testosterone as we hit a certain age. At what age do most men's bodies begin producing less testosterone? Take a wild guess. Don't cheat.

Thirty.

The same age I was at this point in my story.

My body had begun setting a future trap for me. Glucose production was ramping up, and since I wasn't burning it, sugar was being stored as fat. And not only that, but estrogen production was also making it harder to maintain my chiseled musculature; there may be a *slight* exaggeration there, but only slight. Remember how us retired military types sometimes tell stories.

In the meantime, estrogen was doing double duty by simultaneously killing off my testosterone soldiers by the thousands, even as it turned out my vaunted testosterone army was deserting me anyway.

I didn't know any of that yet. I was on my club/ Denny's/workout/club thing and living it up. Or pretending to.

I had my body setting a trap for me that I'd fall prey to at some point in the future, but I was none the wiser.

It was time for me to head back to Asia to get married, and even though the trap had been sprung, I was complete-ly unaware of what lay ahead and still feeling like a champ. I was up to the mid-230s by then, and I would end up going to the Philippines several times over the next couple of years while my wife's visa was being processed. At least I was not clubbing any-more, but why does marriage put weight on people?

OK, OK, maybe it's just me.

Or maybe it was that on my trips to the Philip-pines, I'd wake up drinking Tanduay liquor; I blame it on the time zone. Plus, Tanduay was like twenty-five cents a bottle. Now I already told you about liquor and its effects on the body when consumed in excess. I wonder if cheap liquor has an even worse

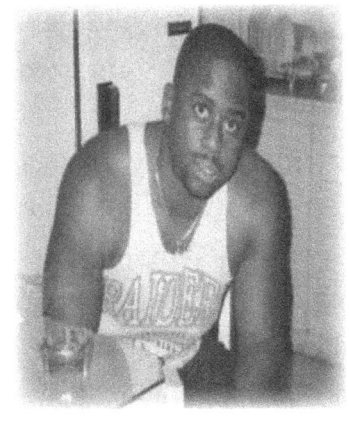

effect? Somehow, I bet it does.

I love ordering room service; I did that a lot in the Philippines too. Because I adore the concept. I lay in the bed, picked up the phone, ordered food, and somebody brought it. And I ate it in bed. Love this—it's a stroke of pure genius.

I loved ordering room service so much, I ordered room service when I wasn't even hungry. Then I lounged in bed, eating like a king with a drumstick in one hand, a shake in the other, before I picked up the phone and bellowed, "Burgers! I must have more burgers!"

That's pretty close to the truth.

Here's something else cool in the mid-'90s Philippines, at least it was to me: most of the Filipinos thought I was a famous American basketball player.

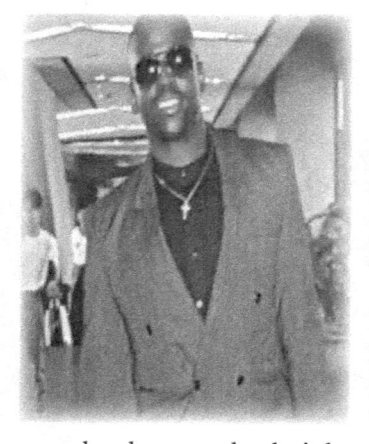

I mean it. There weren't too many Americans running around the Philippines in the '90s, so I literally attracted crowds everywhere I went. I'm only six foot one; that's not short, but definitely not even remotely close to the height of the average basketball player. Regardless, everywhere I went, they yelled out "Shaq O'Neal!" Or they stared. Or they followed me. And they gave me free stuff. As in free food and drink. Star City is an amusement park; when my new wife and I went there, it meant free hot dogs and cotton candy. At the mall? Free Kentucky Fried Chicken. At the restaurants? Free drinks. I suppose they loved the crowds I was attracting, and everyone wanted me to stop and hang out at their spot, so my groupies would stop there too.

Seriously. I had groupies. Paparazzi too. It was kind of fun. I was famous. I was happy my new Filipino in-laws didn't bust me. And why would they? They were getting free stuff too.

Eventually, I told everyone I was a nobody, though. I admitted I was nobody famous, and I was just a regular, average American, a humble serviceman, and I stopped accepting their free food and drinks because I was weary of the deception.

Just kidding. I never stopped. I accepted it all. If they offered it today, I'd accept it right now. Did I mention the crowds, free food, and free drink? I kept frontin'. Who wouldn't?

Because like I said—it was cool.

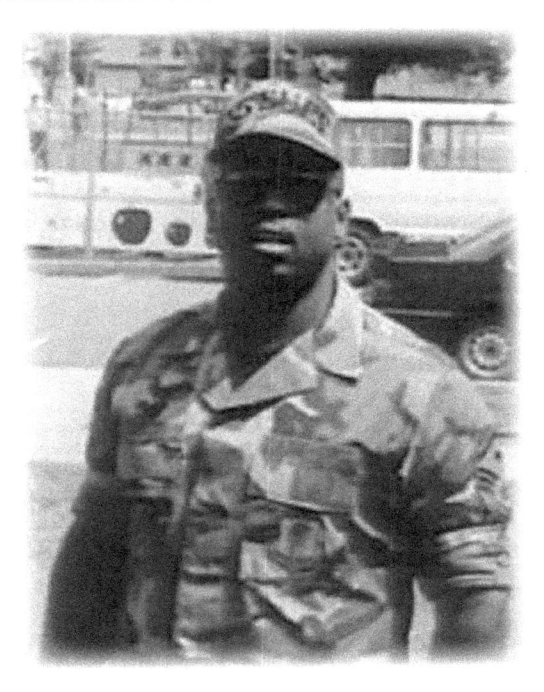

Now my career as an Air Force first sergeant begins. It's a big deal in the military; let me explain what that means.

The first sergeant is on duty twenty-four hours a day, seven days a week, to take care of anything that negatively impacts an airman's health, welfare, morale, discipline, or military readiness; that is true for the airman or their family members. The first sergeant exercises general supervision of all enlisted airmen, represents the commander's priorities and vision to the airmen, and ensures the collective needs of the squadron's airmen and families are communicated back to the commanding officer.

I was selected to serve as a first sergeant when I was thirty-two years old; that's extremely young by Air Force standards, and to be honest, I was honored to be selected for this duty. It made me more than a little nervous, and I took my responsibilities seriously. I said that so I can say this:

I spent the rest of that decade doing things the right way, or trying to. Because first sergeants have to be examples, they can't be all up in the club, drinking all the time, cutting up, and getting free stuff pretending to be a basketball star or allowing people to believe it, which is essentially the same thing, right? They can't be eating everything in sight and letting themselves get out of shape. First sergeants are always on display, front and center; everyone notices you; everyone is watching you 100 percent of the time, so you must do it right. No mistakes allowed.

My heart was in the right place, but even though I was doing the right thing 100 percent of the time, it still didn't quite work for me physically.

I had already permanently left behind the NCO Club and other clubs like it. I didn't miss it at all, but working out was still hard to get to. I typically worked from 7:00 a.m. till 5:00 p.m., but then I never knew when I was going to get called back out to handle an issue for one of my airmen.

Airman fighting with their spouse? Call the first sergeant. Airman in trouble or under arrest? Call the first sergeant. Loud noise complaint in the barracks? Call the first sergeant. Airman depressed or suicidal? Call the first sergeant.

Basically it goes like this: Airman [fill in the blank with whatever you can think of]? Call the first sergeant.

A first sergeant never knows when they will be called, what they might get called out to handle, or how long it will take to stabilize the situation. That's why a first sergeant can't just go home and start working out.

That made working out a sometimes thing. If there were no calls, I wanted to rest. If there were calls, I might not get back home until 10:00 p.m., midnight, or 3:00 in the morning. And some of those calls were stressful; I couldn't come back and have a drink to relax, because I could get called out again. You don't know how many times I'd come back home, then get called right back out again. I couldn't work out for stress relief. Oh, I got it in sometimes, but like I said, you never knew. The first sergeant is human, and human beings need to relax sometimes; what could I possibly do for stress relief?

Wait, I know—go back to that winning philosophy that had served me so well since my didn't-really-go-to-college days:

When in doubt…eat.

In the military, you have to pass a fitness test every year, which is not necessarily easy if you imagine coming home late, hungry, and stressed and just diving into some peanut butter and jelly, then crashing into bed. Not healthy either, is it? How about catching some fast food on the run, wolfing it down, and getting back to work? Or skipping meals due to being so busy, then eating three times more than what is necessary to catch up?

I did well enough to pass my annual fitness evaluations, though; I did everything possible to try to stay on top of things, and a couple of years, it was close but I never failed, which would have been extremely embarrassing. Somehow I managed to squeak by and pass my fitness test every year.

I had turned thirty-nine when I was reassigned to my toughest first sergeant assignment yet: the 311th Training Squadron at the Presidio of Monterey, California. There were about eleven hundred brand-new airmen in long, demanding language training. This was my fifth squadron as a first sergeant and, by size alone, put all my previous four squadrons together and the 311th was bigger than those squadrons combined. And they were all new to the Air Force, right out of basic training.

It is much harder to lead and care for new, inexperienced airmen.

And not only that, but these airmen were also extremely intelligent; they were all specially recruited and had to be supersmart to get selected for language training. From a first sergeant's perspective, the issue is that smart people will test limits in ingenious ways if they're not challenged. I don't intend any disrespect, but there are times when I think a person can be *too* smart for the military. I mean, there were times I wanted to scream, "Stop questioning everything and *do what I tell you, or I'm going to drag your intelligent, battered carcass all over this [bleep-bleep] post!*"

I'm pretty sure I did repeat that phrase or others like it a few thousand times at a very intense volume.

In any case, the decade was closing; I was approaching forty, and I was up to 248 pounds. Who knew I would ever be that close to 250? I had tried everything I used to do fitness-wise, but I was still up twenty pounds that decade. That's only two pounds a year; it creeps up slowly, doesn't it? You don't even recognize it. To be sure, it crept up on me so slowly, I never saw it coming. It was like food was doing drivebys on me. Combine that with the fact that I was still passing all my annual fitness evaluations, and it's no surprise nobody told me I was fat.

CHAPTER 4

SKINTIGHT

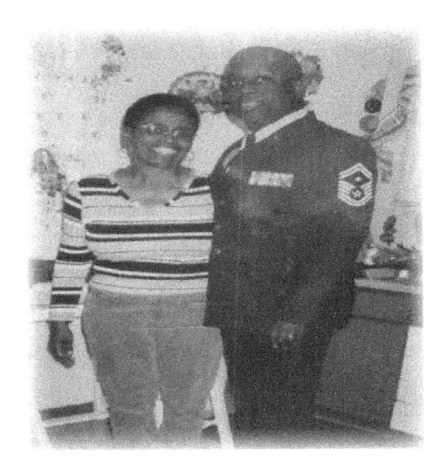

LIKE I SAID in the last chapter, that training squadron in Monterey was tough. I'd turned forty years old, and for the first time, I was getting a little bit sensitive about my weight. I'll give you an example: it's a training squadron, so since the airmen were still young in their military careers, they had to do things like march in parades. As their first sergeant, I was supposed to march with them. Well, after one of our parade marches, I was up in the stands, and I overheard two young officers talking. And one officer says to the other, "Did you see that Air Force first sergeant? That dude is as big as a house." I thought two things when I heard that—first I thought, "Do they not see me? I'm standing right *here*." That thought was rapidly replaced by another, more sobering reality: they were calling me fat. There could be no more denying it. I was, as they said, as big as a house. They were right too. I could feel it. And if those two young officers saw it, everyone who was watching the parade saw the same thing. The knowledge was a little humiliating, so hearing what they were saying about me gave birth to a solemn vow, one I swore I would keep.

You probably think I vowed I would get in shape or eat right or something like that, huh? No, that would be honorable, but that wasn't my vow.

I vowed that I wouldn't march in any more parades. Ever.

And I kept that vow. I delegated that honor to my subordinates. No more marching in parades for me. Not because I was insulted or even worried. Because over time, I decided they weren't calling me fat; I decided they were admiring my massive, chiseled physique, and they were wishing they could be like me.

The mind is a powerful weapon, isn't it?

Nevertheless, the struggle had begun in earnest. I'd decided that no one had told me I was fat. I hadn't even told myself I was fat. I didn't have to, but deep down, I knew it. And I was scrambling hard to do something about it, but no matter how hard I tried, I could still feel myself failing.

Have you ever had that feeling? That feeling of putting your absolute all into something but still feeling yourself failing as victory slowly slips away?

It sucks.

I started hitting the gym harder than I ever had before, but I've never really been a big fan of gyms. I needed the gym when I was playing football, but my real love is boxing, and that's a sport where apart from the sparring, a lot of the training is individual. I'm not a huge fan of gyms, because they're too crowded; remember my introvert thing from the club scene? It was still a thing with me. It still is, even today. I want to do what I want to do when I want to do it and for as long as I feel like doing it. I don't want to wait, I don't want to rush, I don't want to be asked to spot fellow workout enthusiasts, and I don't want to converse. I never thought I could hit my stride in the gym. And not only that, but at a training base like the Presidio, I was also the first sergeant, the second-ranking enlisted Airman on the entire post. When I walked into the gym, it was always "all eyes on me." I wanted to yell, "What are y'all looking at? I ain't Tupac! I just wanna work out! Mind your own dang business…" It's easy to see why the gym never really worked out that well for me.

I decided to try some jogging. Nice, solitary jogging; throw some music in the earphones and take a peaceful morning jog. It was kind of cool, but eventually I found out that was one of the problems; Monterey mornings were more than cool—Monterey mornings were cold. Really cold. And running in the cold isn't fun. I could put on gear that kept me warm, but that wasn't comfortable to run in. Maybe I could have handled the cold, but what I truly didn't like were the animals. I'm usually an animal lover, but…those deer were scary. They would be perfectly still, then jump out when you got too close. Now deer don't bite, but those raccoons that roam the post? They were fearless. They didn't give ground either.

They'd attack. And they were fast too. But what was as bad as the scary wildlife was that I lived in the middle of a hill. Running up a hill is a big problem for obvious reasons, but running down a hill is also a big negative because you know the uphill run is coming. You have to run home sometime, right?

Jogging didn't last too long either.

Now no one was calling me fat, but I knew I needed to do something. I had achieved a high military rank, which is good, but the more rank you have, the more visible you are; makes sense, right? And add to that, my job as a first sergeant was to *enforce* standards, not be a walking model for how people were *not* supposed to look. Plus, high-ranking first sergeants had a responsibility to mentor and develop younger NCOs too.

The result was that I dived into every dieting craze that came along, and let me tell you—*none* of it worked for me.

I tried the Atkins diet. That's the diet where you eat low carbohydrates, but that diet pointed out some essential truths: like, for example, there are a lot of tempting foods that have about a gazillion carbs in them. And worse than that, I don't know if it's just me, but whenever I told my brain it couldn't have something, my brain would almost always respond, "Oh yeah? Well, we'll just see about that." Then my brain would remind me of my food playboy tendencies and make me crave carbs like real playboys crave…ummm…you know.

I told you: the mind is a powerful weapon.

I tried something called the "Seven-Day Color Diet," which entailed eating different-colored foods every day. It's supposed to ensure you're getting a balanced diet.

Day 1, I ate white foods. Day 2 was red food day, and so on and so forth. Well, the first problem was that on most days, I completely forgot what color food I was supposed to be eating.

Secondly, they had an Orange Food Day in the diet. Orange food. Really? Think about it: what was I supposed to eat on Orange Food Day? Just oranges and carrots? What other foods are orange anyway? Life Savers? Halloween candy?

I don't think I made it seven days. In fact—I only made it up to Orange Food Day. Then, that diet was a wrap. What a stupid idea.

I tried that South Beach Diet thing. I don't remember much except that I couldn't eat any of the foods I liked and at fifteen hundred calories a day; I couldn't even eat enough of the foods I didn't like. Fifteen hundred calories a day was not realistic for a man of my size, so that diet didn't last long. I moved on to join the SlimFast craze instead. Those SlimFast snacks were tasty, but they were kind of expensive, and I found out that just because it says SlimFast on the package doesn't mean you can eat five of them every meal and expect to get slim.

I was trying, though. Trying *really* hard—but no matter what I did, it just wasn't working.

After Monterey, I departed on another overseas tour to Spain—a beautiful country where they really know how to eat.

In Spain we worked on a Spanish air base side by side with the Spanish Air Force, and accordingly, we respected Spanish customs. In Spain, there's breakfast in the morning; then "tapas" midmorning. Think of tapas like finger foods, something any food playboy would love, because you can make tapas out of anything. Throw food that you like together, cut it up small, and you've got yourself a tapa. Then, eat them all.

Then there's lunch, and after lunch? The country shuts down for three hours for a siesta. Seriously. We had to shut down too. We couldn't fly jets around Spanish airspace when they were siesta-ing, right? Besides, we partnered up with our Spanish teammates on air traffic control and aircraft maintenance. So we couldn't fly; when they went on siesta, we did too.

At about 4:30 or so, siesta was over, and it was time for the predinner meal. Nothing is open, but the entire country erupts with activity again around 8:00 p.m. until midnight for dinner.

In short, I ate around the clock.

And by late 2004, my weight was up to 268 pounds.

It was when I was promoted to Chief Master Sergeant the following year that I unknowingly started a weight yo-yo that would last for over a decade.

In the Air Force, Chief Master Sergeant is the absolute highest enlisted rank; there is no higher rank possible for an enlisted airman. Only 1 percent of the enlisted force can wear the rank; it is a huge career accomplishment that most service members will never attain. It is a rank that, once achieved, is a lifetime term of address. Kind of like boxers who get called "Champ" even after they've lost the title or retired. Or like a president who is always addressed as "Mr. President" (someday, "Madam President," I'm sure). Being promoted to Chief Master Sergeant is an extremely significant accomplishment.

I was borderline embarrassed, though. No one was saying anything to me about my weight, because I suppose I was carrying my weight well, but at 270 pounds, I knew I was too heavy. In fact, I knew I was fat, but it felt like there was nothing I could do; no matter what I tried, it was as if I was doomed to failure again.

I started counting calories around this point. I worked out in every way I possibly could. I ran, rode the stationary bike, did the stationary mountain-climber thing, took step aerobics class in the gym, lifted free weights, did the Nautilus; I tried everything to the point where trying to stay in shape just to keep from humiliating myself became my all-consuming task.

I say I had to keep from humiliating myself because now, in my mind, I imagined everyone was talking about me. I imagined everyone was laughing at the new, big, fat Chief, wondering how that guy passed his fitness exams, and questioning why he got promoted.

I told you before and I'll tell you again—the mind is a powerful weapon.

By the time I returned stateside, to Arizona, my efforts had paid off somewhat, and my weight was down to 258 pounds.

I should have known it wouldn't last.

You see, the problem was that I could lose a little or at least not gain if I kept up calorie counting and a hard workout routine, but my routine was not sustainable; if I stopped for even a week, I'd gain weight back, and it was even harder to lose it when I buckled down to business to try to lose again.

I knew, because six months after I arrived at my Arizona Air Force Base, my weight was all the way up to 274—my highest weight ever to that point.

It was stressful. And stress is bad for weight loss. In addition to triggering that emotional eating response in some people, stress also produces cortisol.

That's the hormone that produces body fat, especially around the gut.

Gaining weight, combined with stress, also increased my blood pressure to dangerous levels. Now get this—I went to the doctor for some meds to lower my blood pressure, and to be honest, I don't remember too much of what he said, but I definitely remember two things: first, he prescribed me a "beta blocker," and then he went on to explain how it worked, but I didn't listen to a single word. He was going on and on, but I got the gist of it: take this pill, blood pressure goes down.

I heard that clearly. I mean, I'm not an idiot.

I also heard clearly when the doctor said one of the side effects could be weight gain.

I stared at this doctor like he had three heads. I was literally speechless. With the battle I was fighting? I didn't need any help whatsoever gaining weight.

I never took that medicine. Not a single pill until the day I retired from the military.

Instead, I just worked out harder and counted calories tighter. And five months later, I had battled my way back down to 260 pounds.

Again.

Of course, it didn't last. It never did.

The struggle was too intense, more difficult every day. It was impossible to sustain for long and, despite my absolute best efforts, over the next year, my weight crept back up to 270.

Then a year later—280.

I felt powerless to do anything to stop my weight gain; it was avalanching me now. I thought it was incredible that I passed all my fitness tests, and no one noticed how huge I was. That time in my life was extremely stressful, the most stressful period of my life to date. I was waiting to be found out as a fraud, waiting for the military to tell me I was no longer meeting standards. In the military, if you can't meet your weight standard, they will take your rank away and keep taking it away until you meet standards. I seriously considered retiring from the military simply because I couldn't meet the weight standard anymore.

I was waiting to be fired. Instead, I got promoted.

The Command Chief Master Sergeant is the senior enlisted Airman on the base, responsible for several thousand service members and their families, and the primary adviser to the base commander on

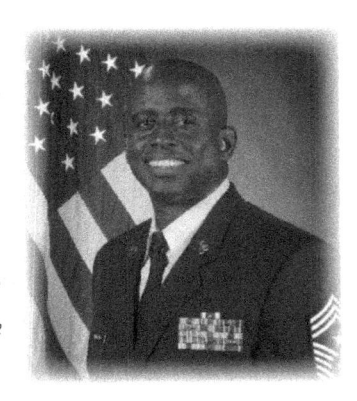

all matters pertaining to enlisted airmen. I already told you how prestigious it was to earn Chief Master Sergeant rank. Command Chief Master Sergeant is the best of *those* distinguished leaders.

And the base commander wanted *me*.

I couldn't believe it. The selection didn't stress me out, though. Not at all. It did the opposite. It calmed me down.

My thought was "Hey, maybe I'm not so fat. The colonel could have picked any Chief, but he picked *me*. He wouldn't pick a fat slob for this job, so I must be legit."

I relaxed. And guess what?

I lost weight.

Remember that. I *relaxed*...then I lost weight.

It'll work for you too.

I was doing the same thing I was doing before, and eight months into my job, I was all the way back down to 253. Now granted, I was up at 4:00 a.m. to work out. I guess the weight loss felt good to me, so

I wanted to keep it going. There were times I would delegate one of my many meetings to another Chief or to a first sergeant so I could take off for a run around the base. Those runs would be anywhere from three to ten miles.

By November 2011, my weight was back down to 244. I hadn't weighed in that low since my late thirties, about ten years before, and it...felt...fantastic.

Too bad it wouldn't last.

It was around that time that I had consistent blood pressure readings of around 190 over 120.

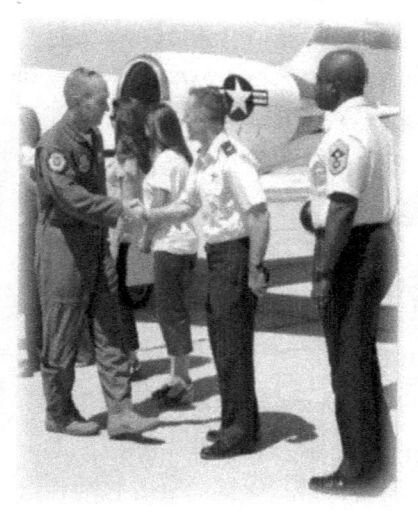 That's crisis territory. The military doctors would keep prescribing me beta blockers that I wouldn't take, but I lied and told the doctors I was taking them. When they "didn't work," they'd increase the dosage. I resisted taking any blood pressure meds,

but once my blood pressure got that high, exercise was out. *Every* exercise was out. I could "feel" my heart even just walking or sitting. And I'm going to be very honest right now.

I didn't want to die.

But I still wouldn't take the meds.

Was not being fat *that* important? Worth risking my life over? Clearly, it wasn't. I should have been taking my meds all along. And if you're on some meds with a potential weight gain side effect, *who cares?* Take your meds. I mean it. And do it today. Then keep doing it from now on. I'm being absolutely serious: *take your meds.*

But me? Since I couldn't exercise anymore, nine months later when I reached mandatory retirement from active duty, I was back up to 257. I risked my health for nothing. I gained weight anyway and was highly annoyed.

I was relieved to retire, though. As challenging as the military was, my hardest battle, the toughest thing of all for the past several years, by far, had been my own internal battle. Now I had no more worries; I was out. No one could judge me anymore. I could hide out. I could relax. And finally—I started taking my blood pressure meds.

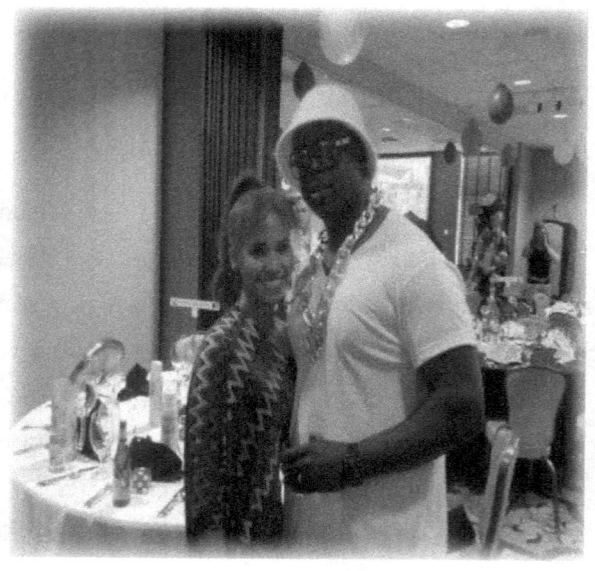

I celebrated my new freedom by smoking lots of cigars. This was not good for my blood pressure—another dumb, dangerous practice of mine I do not want you to emulate.

And drinking was a part of my freedom celebration. I started most days at noon; I didn't want to drink in the morning, because in my mind, that would have meant I had a problem. And of course, I lived my lifelong philosophy: "When in doubt...eat."

All of it was worse than ever before, because once I retired, I no longer knew my purpose. I was forty-nine years old, and for the past thirty-one years, I had known my 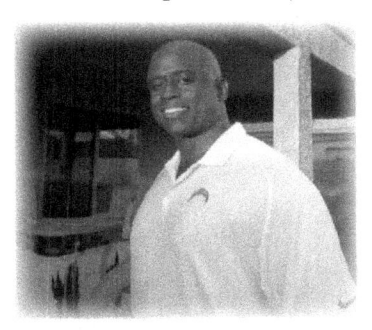 place, my role, where I was going, what I was supposed to be doing, how to do it, and what my identity was. I had known where I fit in, but all of a sudden, there was nothing. I was more than a little bit lost. Eventually, I filled up the nothing I felt inside me with something. I know you know what the something was.

Food. Also alcohol and nicotine. But mostly food. Maybe I couldn't drink until noon, but I could eat as soon as my eyes opened. And that's what I did.

And within four months of retiring and by the end of the decade, I had gained back nearly twenty-five pounds, and my weight matched my lifetime high of 280 pounds.

I gained thirty-two pounds during the decade.

But since I was retired from the military, at least there was no one around to tell me I was fat.

CHAPTER 5

SLIPPIN' INTO
DARKNESS

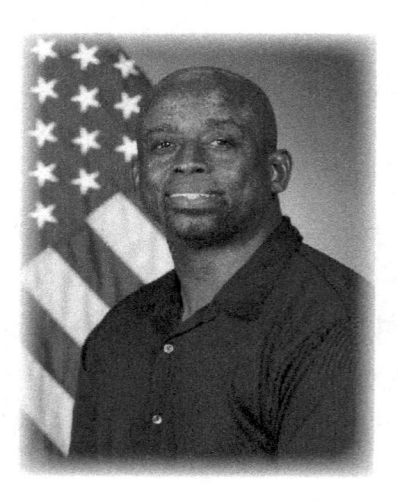

A NEW DECADE began. I was stressed out for a while, trying to figure out what I was going to do next, but the year I turned fifty, I also started a new postmilitary career. It was a very good job, and I was lucky to get a position that once again provided me with purpose. I got hired to be the manager for the resilience program and comprehensive wellness initiatives on a military base. It's also the year I got diagnosed with having a tumor on my adrenal gland. Kind of shook me up a little bit, but turned out it was benign. Nevertheless, it still caused problems. Benign adrenal tumors may be noncancerous, but they overproduce cortisol. Here we go again—the stupid hormone that leads to weight gain.

Does *everything* increase cortisol production? Because it sure seemed that way.

So at this point in the story, I was thinking, "this is some bullshit."

I know, I know. It's profanity. It's the only word of profanity in this entire book. That's pretty good for a thirty-year military veteran; most of us tend to cuss a lot. I struggled mightily to try to come up with a different word, but as it turns out, it's the only word that fit the situation because I was sincerely mad at my life.

Because it really was some damn, stupid bullshit.

That's why I decided to live with a single word of profanity in this book.

OK...two words. Three profane words if you consider "damn" a term of profanity.

It didn't seem fair, though.

I was still working out and trying to at least maintain my weight since, in my own mind, clearly I was doomed to be heavy. Nobody was calling me fat, though, and I wasn't saying it to myself either. I was heavy. Not fat.

But man, was I heavy.

Two years after starting my new job, I was up to 290 pounds. I got one of those scales that measured

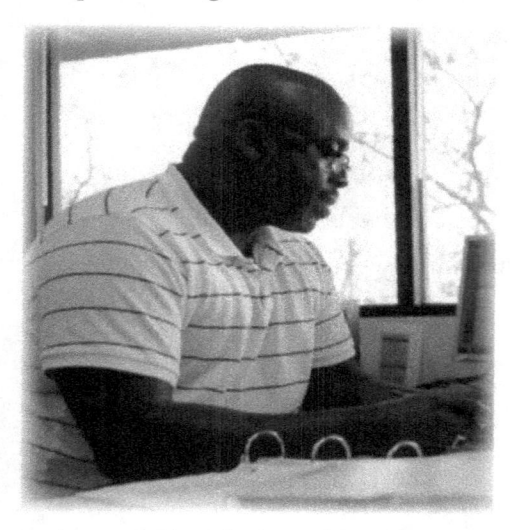

body fat percentage; I figured, "OK, so I'm heavy—but I'm muscular, right? That's what everybody says." A body fat scale would legitimize where I was physically, put me at around the 20 percent or 25 percent body fat that was expected for my age, then I could go back to living my beautifully crafted life philosophy.

Not so fast.

My body fat was 42 percent.

Almost half of my body was pure fat.

Believe it or not, I shrugged it off. I blamed it on the adrenal thing. I thought, "Hey, it's not my fault my stupid glands are flooding my old, muscular, but heavy body with hormones." Still though—gaining ten pounds in two years? Let's do that math: gaining ten pounds in two years would be a fifty-pound gain in ten years if things kept going the way they were going. And an extra fifty pounds by the time I was sixty would have me weighing…wow. And what would I look like when my body fat percentage went *over* 50 percent?

I felt powerless to stop it. Have you ever felt like that? Once again, it seemed seared into my very being: "I know I'm getting ready to lose, it's going to suck badly, it's going to hurt me physically, mentally, spiritually, and socially, but there is absolutely nothing I can do to stop it."

I hate that feeling.

I bet you do too. Unfortunately, I was right. I was getting ready to hit rock bottom.

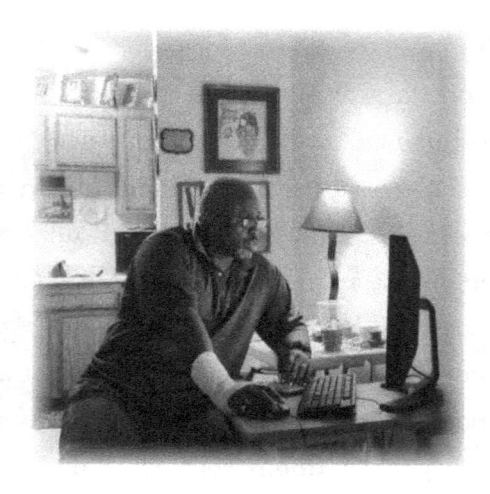

Over the next year, I picked up nine more pounds. I remember the day I weighed 299 pounds. I was at an appointment with my cardiologist; I stepped on the scale, and the nurse wrote it down in my record. I watched her write it down, and as I considered my situation, I made a silent vow. Just like the vow I made when the two officers admired me for being as big as a house, it was a vow that I intended to keep forever. Solemn vows are like that. They're serious business.

I vowed that day to never step on or look at another scale.

I knew I was going to go over three hundred pounds; it was inevitable and when the day came, I didn't want to know even though I already knew. My pant size was forty-six inches. In the waist. I could get away with a forty-four or a forty-two-inch waist if the pants weren't too stiff; I wore them low, I sucked in my belly, and I wore a bigger shirt.

The thing is, it was so obvious I was getting even heavier. I could feel it. I kept my vow and refused to get on a scale for any reason. I also refused to take pictures. I didn't want to take pictures with my wife. I didn't want to take pictures with my children. I bet you know why. The camera doesn't lie.

Stupid camera.

My guess is my weight got up to about 320.

No pictures exist of me during that time in my life.

But I'm a fighter. In my mind and my spirit, I am a fighter. And fighters fight—it's what we do. A fighter trains to be mindful; a fighter trains to cover up when getting battered, or even take a knee, if necessary. A fighter trains to listen for their corner when the opponent has temporarily turned the lights off so that the corner can tell the fighter, "You're OK; listen for our voices, and we will bring you back. We will lead you home."

It's a mental thing, and I'm going to admit, that fighter's mentality came in handy, because I fought back against some extremely dark thoughts during those days. It was bad. I fought back hard against a lot of negative self-talk where I questioned my own value as a human being. I fought back against intense feelings of shame, self-loathing, and even self-hatred that threatened to overwhelm every good or positive thing I had ever done in my entire life. I fought back against a near constant barrage of thoughts such as "Nobody lives forever, so I'm going to enjoy myself. I don't care anymore."

Except I wasn't enjoying myself. I was lying to myself, and I had stopped believing my lies.

I continued to battle mentally against a powerful urge to stay out of sight, eat more since I was doomed to fail anyway, and just surrender on the whole deal. Giving in seemed like it would be so much easier; there wouldn't be any more stress. I imagined myself at four hundred pounds, unable to walk or get out of bed and not caring about either…but I fought it.

I wanted life to just leave me alone and let me be. It was hard. It was the most difficult time of my life. I almost gave up.

But fighters fight.

It was an up-and-down battle, but I kept fighting, and when I was sure I was not over three hundred, I broke my vow and got back on a scale.

Can you imagine being happy to weigh "only" 275 pounds? My guess is my weight had gone up to 320 or so, so my fight had resulted in a forty- or fifty-pound weight loss, even though I still lost my breath standing up. I enjoyed the moment. Experience had taught me my weight would eventually yo-yo up again, but I allowed myself to enjoy the temporary victory.

Then I came upon something new. Something I hadn't heard of before.

I was visiting some friends and sitting, having my normal afternoon cocktail—Crown Royal on the rocks. I was up to drinking water glasses full of alcohol back then but not getting drunk. OK, maybe I was getting a little drunk. That's not good. Clearly, I was not out of the woods just yet.

I was sitting on their couch, drinking and chatting, and while I was doing that, they were walking in circles around their living room while they chatted. Sometimes they would break into a little jog. Sometimes they would stop and chat and jog in place. I finally asked them what they were doing.

They explained they were "getting steps."

Then they showed me their step trackers and broke down the whole science of steps. Ten thousand steps a day for a healthy heart. A minimum of 250 steps an hour during the waking hours. Then they explained they were in these challenges with other family members on social media to see who could win their group step challenges.

I found it all kind of amusing. Then I looked at them both, and a thought occurred to me.

What they were doing was working.

When I got home, I bought myself a fitness watch and got to steppin' myself! And starting late summer 2016, I began tracking my steps. I got twenty-three thousand steps that day...and so it began.

I got into counting my steps. It felt different. I researched it, and it made sense to me. Within a month I hit forty thousand steps for the first time, and my weight had dropped to 265.

I thought maybe this time it would last.

Let me explain something. You probably know this, but getting that many steps in a day is hard. Really hard. OK, it's not that hard; it's just walking. Or jogging in place. But it takes a long, *long* time. It's not like working out in the gym for an hour and being done for the day. It's waking up and walking. It's walking to meetings at work. It's walking during breaks. It's walking while watching television. It's walking until it's time for bed. I used to go out on my back porch to smoke cigars, drink, and listen to my beloved old-school music. I called it "Club Howard." Well, I still went to Club Howard nightly, but I grabbed steps while I reminisced to my old-school music, puffed cigars, and drank liquor.

And some of those old school jams made my steppin' a little livelier. Put on some "Dusic," by Brick, or a little "Knee Deep," and you'll step like a champion too. Or maybe it was the alcohol. Whatever. A step is a step, right?

I probably looked like an idiot.

I didn't care. I wasn't in the gym, so I only looked like an idiot to my family, but my step routine was working. For the first time in years, *something* was working.

By the end of the year, four months after I started, I hit fifty thousand steps in a single day for the first time.

I picked up the pace.

A few months into the new year, I set a personal record of 247,000 steps for the week, but even more impressively, my weight was all the way down to 255. This was just about the same weight I had been when I'd retired from active duty. I had been annoyed to be in the 250s when I retired, but when I saw the 250s again five years later?

Pure joy.

I picked up the pace even further.

I set a record of sixty thousand steps in a single day. I obliterated my weekly record when, one week, I recorded 273,000 steps. What helped were the step challenges I was in with other step fanatics from all over the world. There'd be a group of ten people online: that housewife from Chicago…the casino guy from Las Vegas…that realtor from Texas…all of those people and more, random people, all coming together online to push each other to get more steps, provide encouragement and humor. I was really into the step thing.

When I set a new personal record of seventy thousand steps in a single day, my feet were literally bleeding by the end of the day. They didn't hurt, though, and you know why? Because winning doesn't hurt. Winning feels sweet. I saw victory coming, and the thought of it pushed any pain out of mind. The time I had to dedicate to my stepping efforts was likewise irrelevant. I was laser focused on the victory I knew was coming.

And then, out of nowhere, it stopped working.

I don't know why. I was still stepping hard. I'd walk high up into the Arizona mountains—I'd take a big stick or pick up a rock along the way, because there are wild animals up there. Stray dogs too. I didn't want to hurt any animals, but I didn't want to get eaten or bitten either. There were some nice walks up there, though, and it was peaceful; I could look down on the entire city. It was about ten miles round trip.

But it still didn't work anymore.

I had another route. Walking along the highway. There's a long stretch of Arizona desert highway between my house and civilization, and I'd walk it. No need for weapons on this one. People would honk encouraging greetings to me sometimes. That highway got hot sometimes, though; a few times I walked so far, I got sunstroke or sun drunk or sun *something*.

I'd be so hot, pouring sweat; I'd find myself walking in the middle of the highway with no recollection of why I was walking in the middle of the highway. I'd call my wife to come pick me up on those days, sweat pouring off of me, feeling completely drained.

But it still didn't work anymore.

I kept doing it, but I couldn't figure out why I was gaining weight again. By October 2017, I was back up to 265, and my fifty-fourth birthday saw me at 278.

Again.

And that's where my weight remained, no matter what I did.

I wasn't disappointed. I wasn't mad either. I wasn't anything. Because I had known all along it was coming. I accepted it.

Again.

I had just turned fifty-four, and it seemed like I had been fighting this battle for a lifetime. To be honest, once again, I was tired of fighting it. I kept doing my step thing, because for one thing, I was used to it, and if I wasn't going to do that, then what? For another, one of the step partners in the group I was in presented a challenge to me that I had never done.

One hundred thousand steps. In one day.

I still wasn't losing weight, but if I stayed at it, who knew if it wouldn't start working again?

One hundred thousand steps. In one day.

We decided December 26 would be the day. This was going to take some planning. A person can quick-step about eight thousand steps an hour, so one

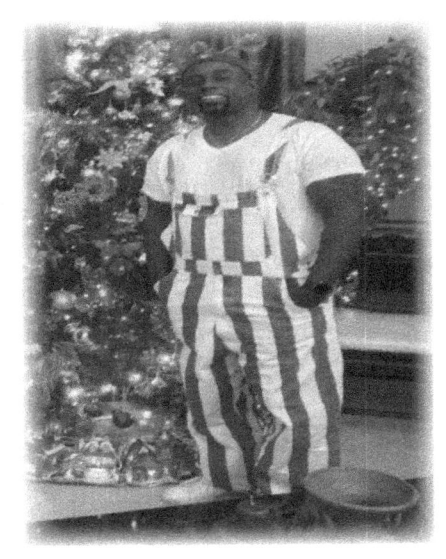

hundred thousand steps was possible with twelve hours of stepping. That's twelve hours. Straight. That's hard. Plus, a person must eat, go to the bathroom, and rest. I figured I could wake up at midnight and grab the first twenty-five thousand. Then rest. By the time I woke up, I'd plan for five thousand steps an hour for fifteen hours, from 8:00 a.m. to 11:00 p.m. with fifteen-minute breaks every hour. Then I'd make it with an hour to spare.

Basically, it's walking or running in place for fifteen hours. Sound easy?

I woke up at 1:00 a.m. already tired. *Everyone* is tired at 1:00 a.m., aren't they? Even so, I got to stepping; that first twenty-five thousand steps took longer than I thought, and it was after 5:00 a.m. when I got back into bed, doubting that I could make it. I was too tired.

I woke up at 8:00 a.m. A little late, but I figured I'd step through a few breaks to make up for lost time. There I was quick-stepping around my kitchen, through my living room, my garage, outside on my back patio, then inside again, quick-stepping around my house like a maniac.

You should have seen how my dog was looking at me. Didn't I tell you in chapter 1 that I was a weirdo that you might not want to copy?

Told you. Hold on, though. Just wait until the next chapter. There's more.

By 7:00 p.m. I had passed my old step record and reached eighty-thousand steps. Five hours left to midnight and twenty thousand steps to go. I rested for a half hour, because at this point, I knew there was no stopping me.

By 10:00 p.m. I had ten thousand steps to go; that many steps normally takes about seventy-five minutes of quick-stepping, so I decided from that point, I'd quick-step all the way to my goal. I poured some drinks to celebrate while I stepped off that last ten thousand steps, which is about four miles.

What a weirdo.

In any case, I made those one hundred thousand steps with about thirty-five minutes to spare. I was a little tipsy and a lot exhausted, but I celebrated virtually with my online stepping partners before collapsing in my bed.

And it was my last hurrah.

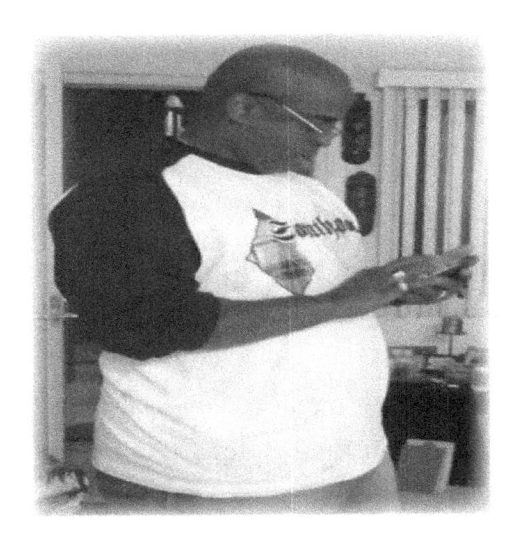

I never even broke thirty thousand steps ever again.

And by March, I'd left my fellow weirdo steppers and had gone back to the normal ten thousand or fifteen thousand per day that reasonable people do.

Looking back, it was as if I knew that I was getting ready to give it up. That stepping took too much time to not be working, but before I gave it up, I wanted to climb that one last step mountain.

And by April of the next year, my weight was back in the 280s.

I had a doctor's appointment in May. I forget what it was for, but I do remember what the doctor said. It was something that no doctor had ever said to me before:

"Do you want to live to see sixty?"

I was shocked. This doctor had a look on her face that I couldn't read. Most doctors at military hospitals loved me. I was retired from active duty, but at my rank, like I said before, you never lose it. I'd always be "Command Chief Howard"; your retired rank is even in your medical records. My picture was still on the wall in the headquarters building. Most doctors would say things to me like "Well, Command Chief, you're looking fairly good. You clearly have a strong base of muscle with a little fat on top, which is to be expected for your age."

I saw later they were actually writing, "Patient is morbidly obese" in my medical record, but they were always verbally gentle.

Until now.

I peered at the little, young doctor who had just challenged the mighty Command Chief Howard to see if she would again utter the words that no one had dared say to me in my fifty-six years on the planet.

And the doctor peered back, waiting for an answer to her question.

When no answer came, the doctor continued, "Well, if you do, you're going to have to make some changes. Even if you survive to see sixty, you may have to say goodbye to your feet if you continue on this path."

Her look said it all. If I continued, she was saying either my worsening diabetes could result in amputation, or maybe she was saying that my stomach would grow so big, I wouldn't be able to see my feet anymore.

Neither option was that attractive.

I thought she was going to say it, but the doctor never actually called me fat. She said something else, though—something that I'd never heard before:

"Have you ever considered intermittent fasting?"

CHAPTER 6

STARTING ALL OVER AGAIN

"FASTING? YOU MEAN as in not eating?"

"That's exactly what I mean."

I stared. Then I stared some more. I didn't need to answer, because the answer was written all over my face.

I'm a food playboy, Doc. Got it? Not gonna happen.

My brave doctor read my refusal clearly and smiled. I was thinking, "What is it with this youngster? She looks like she's been in the military all of five minutes. She acts like she doesn't realize she's talking to the great and powerful Command Chief Master Sergeant Howard.

She wasn't advising a Command Chief though. She was only trying to advise aging, morbidly obese, diabetic, soon-to-be-footless Vince. I told you a few chapters ago, though, the mind is a powerful thing.

"Tell me this: How would you feel going twelve hours without eating if it included the time you were sleeping?"

I considered what she'd just said.

That meant if I stopped eating at 8:00 p.m., could I not eat again until 8:00 a.m. the next day? Is that what she was proposing?

I'm a playboy. The food kind. But I thought I *might* be able to do that if that's what fasting was.

Maybe.

The thing is, I loved eating at night too. Sometimes I would "sleep eat." Some people talk in their sleep. Some sleepwalk. I would "sleep eat." I don't know why. I'd wake up in the middle of the night, go grab some cookies, then head back to bed. Or I might wake up, groggily pour some cereal, eat it, then sleep. Sometimes I'd make a peanut butter and jelly sandwich, wolf it down with some cold milk, then back to bed I'd go.

And often, believe it or not, I'd remember none of it the next day.

There'd be dishes in the sink or crumbs on the counter or a knife with drying peanut butter on it lying around. Sometimes I'd even accidentally leave the cereal box open or would forget to close the bread back up. My wife would get up in the morning and ask me, "Did you eat last night?"

I'd look her right in her face with my biggest, most honest-looking eyes and say, "Nope."

When you're lying, say as few words as possible.

But you know how that other kind of playboy gets caught in the act? With a phone number in the pocket? Or gets overheard on the phone? Or maybe they were spotted with the person they were not supposed to be seeing? Then, when confronted, they respond, "Wasn't me. Looked like me. Sounded like me. Wasn't me, though. You made a mistake."

That was me. But with food: "I know you see the crumbs. The dishes in the sink. The dirty knife. I know my breath still smells like peanut butter. Ignore the tasty morsels still resting on the corner of my mouth."

I'd add, "Wasn't me. Looked like me. Sounded like me. Wasn't me, though. You made a mistake."

Food playboy.

I considered what the doc had said, because I was still kind of stuck on not having any feet in the future. I thought to myself that maybe this fasting thing wasn't that difficult, and I considered giving it a shot.

My little female Doogie Howser gave me all these pamphlets and recommended a book on the benefits of intermittent fasting. I was trying to pay attention, but she could have saved the paper; doing all that research is not my way. That's details—and I don't do details.

It was like teaching myself to play the piano after I retired from the military. I'd always wanted to learn to play piano, so after I retired and had more time on my hands, I got these books and looked at these videos from YouTube, but that was taking too long. I thought, "Hey, I don't want to read music; I don't want to learn about beats, counts, notes, tempo, musical theory, or any of that mess—I just wanna play the ding-dang piano."

Then I just banged away at the keys until I could play a song I could recognize. And it worked.

Intermittent fasting was the same way. I didn't want to read about science and all that. I just wanted to get the basics down and I'd figure out the rest.

And that's what I did.

I started a twelve-hour fast that night. I stopped eating at 7:00 p.m. and committed to not eating or drinking anything but water and black coffee until 7:00 a.m.

It was easy. And as I read about it over time, the science turned out to be interesting.

It turns out everything we eat causes our bodies to produce insulin. *Everything.* Even healthy food like celery produces an insulin response. Even zero-calorie food with artificial sweeteners, like diet soda or Splenda, cause an insulin response. Think of that insulin as sugar, just like the glucose I told you about earlier. So even though the calories are low, this sugary insulin stuff inside our bodies is hard to burn. We can burn calories off by exercising, but that insulin in our bodies? Nope. It doesn't burn away that easy.

And when we don't burn off the insulin, our bodies store it. And how does the body store unburned insulin?

Yep. As fat. Just like glucose.

But what *does* burn the insulin is time. If our bodies don't get insulin from food for twelve hours, the body starts burning off insulin inside like a furnace. And *that* is intermittent fasting. It takes twelve hours of not eating to fire up the body furnace, but every second past twelve hours, our bodies are burning that insulin-sugar for energy.

But there's more.

Everyone is different, but around the sixteen- or eighteen-hour mark of fasting, the body starts producing human growth hormone too. Look that up. Because that's some *good* stuff. It's what teenagers produce, and it makes us better able to build muscle. It doesn't just increase our ability to build muscle, but it also increases our bone density. It increases our exercise effectiveness. And it is a high-level fat and insulin burner too. And for adults, it's antiaging.

I told you. It's good stuff.

Now at about the twenty-hour mark? That's when autophagy kicks in. What's that? Imagine a bunch of body inflammation all throughout your body along with weak, diseased cells. And that inflammation is jacking up your immune system and making you look and feel older. If you don't get rid of that internal inflammation and those diseased cells, they eventually damage healthy organs and can lead to a bunch of diseases, including cancer and Alzheimer's. Google it, like I did, if you don't believe me.

Autophagy cleans out those cells and waters down the inflammation. Autophagy is a fasting-induced process where your strong, healthy cells eat up all of the weak, diseased ones. It's an internal body flush; it's like getting all the stupid junk and spyware out of your computer to optimize operations. Autophagy cleans the body out from the inside.

I didn't know any of that when I started. I just started fasting for twelve hours; I wasn't losing any weight, but I knew I just felt *clean* on the inside. I don't really know how to fully describe that *clean* feeling inside. I felt light; I felt healthy; I felt strong; I just felt *clean*. And even though I was still heavy, I loved the *clean* feeling. After a month or two, I decided to move up to fourteen-hour fasts. I was kind of nervous the first time I tried it. I stopped eating at 6:00 p.m., committed to no sleep eating, and held off on breakfast until 8:00 a.m. the next morning.

And I did it. It was easy.

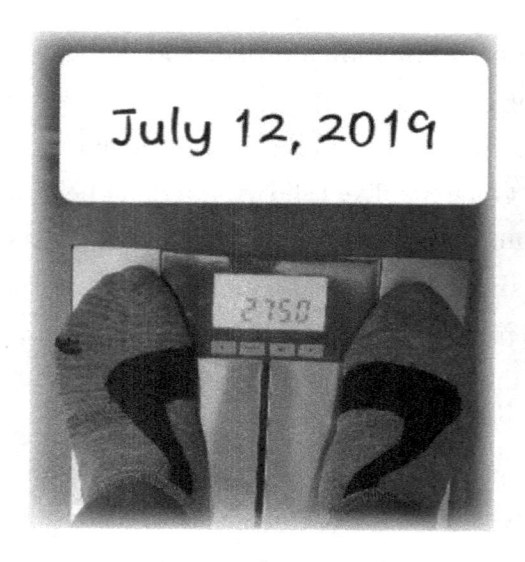

I weighed 275 pounds when I started intermittent fasting but I enjoyed the *clean* I was feeling inside. I had given up on the whole weight loss thing. My body had already broken my heart too many times, so my attitude was "Forget you, Body! Keep your stupid pounds; make me as heavy as you want. I'm getting *clean* inside, OK? I don't care what you do with the pounds anymore."

And I meant it.

But even so, I started losing weight.

A lot.

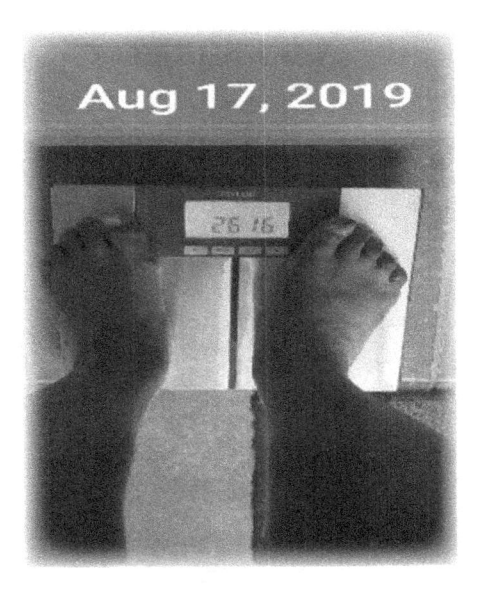

I was 275 pounds when I got on my scale in July 2019, but by August? I was down to 262. I thought that was kind of crazy—thirteen pounds off in a month? No way, Body. Not buying it. I'd been there before, so I refused to get hyped and start souping myself up. I told my body, "I'm not chasing pounds anymore—so just shut up and don't talk to me. I'm too busy chasing the *clean*."

And then I broke 250. I hadn't been in the 240s for over ten years. It wasn't just that; my blood pressure was down to what it had been twenty years pri-

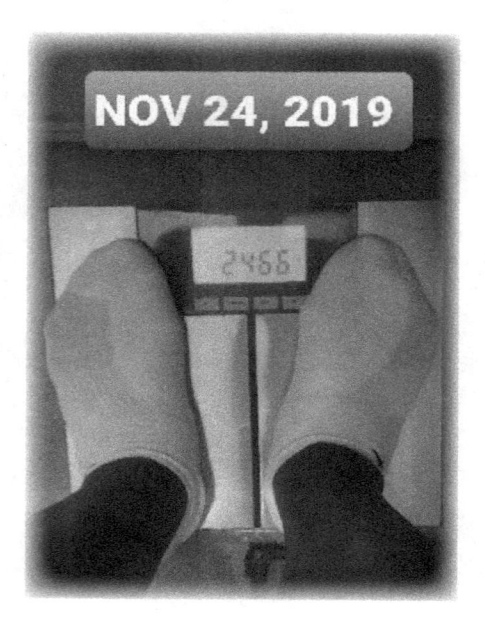

or. So I decided to ramp up my intermittent fasting hours to sixteen hours per day; I stopped eating at 6:00 pm and took in only water and coffee until 10:00 am the next day.

Now I knew I was on to something, but I was not going to chase weight loss. Nope. I still don't care. That's what happens when you get your heart broken too many times, am I right? You stop caring.

Now—why was I taking pictures of my scale? That's a really good question. I had zero idea where

I would end up and had no plans to ever write a book.

I guess I just took the pics and saved them because I'm a weirdo.

A weirdo who kept losing weight.

By the end of the year, I was down to 234. Sorry about the toes. I should have said that before. Diabetes savages the feet, though, and like I said, I didn't know I'd be writing a book. Otherwise, I'd have worn socks all the time.

As I went into the next year, I was down to 215 pounds; that's more than one hundred pounds less than my highest-ever weight. And I'll tell you, now I was feeling myself. I told my body, "I still don't care," and I meant it sincerely; I was all about the process; I was all about the *clean*—but I knew something. And I increased my

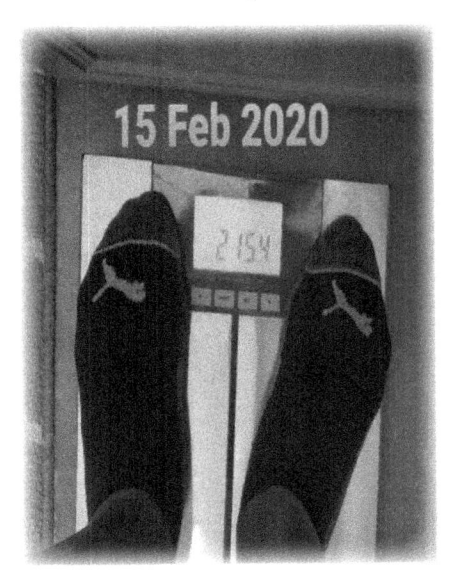

fasting schedule to eighteen hours a day; 6:00 pm to noon the next day.

And when I hit 205 pounds the next month, it occurred to me that I was at a lower weight than I'd been for my first fight *thirty years earlier*.

I could have stopped there, but I didn't know what "stopping" meant; this was my lifestyle now. I was up to fasting twenty hours a day, and I had incorporated it into my personal and professional relationships. Many times in the past, I ate when other people ate. It was a social thing. But now? People ate, and I chatted without eating with them like it was no

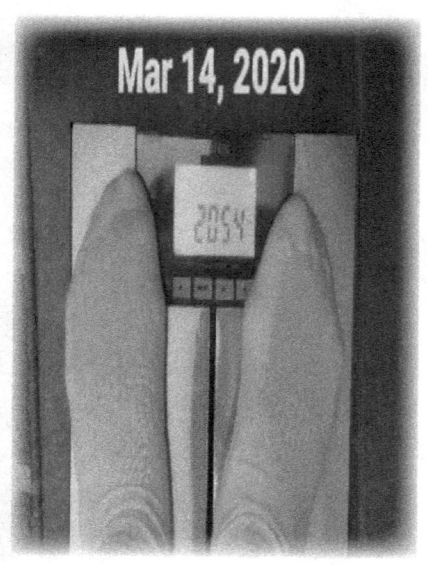

big deal. If I was fasting—no eating. It was a simple rule.

Intermittent fasting led me to another new practice that became a permanent lifestyle change: I didn't eat when I got hungry—I ate *before* I got hungry. In other words, I ate when my brain said the fast was over and it was now time to eat. Waiting to eat until I felt hunger made me more likely to overeat, but eating when it was time to eat made it easier to eat smaller. Now, there was no more waiting until I was hungry. Once the fast ended, I could eat whatever I wanted as long as I counted the calories without cheating. That's how it was; it was the new reality. There were no practices to "stop." This was my life now, so I kept going.

And in May, my weight dipped under two hundred pounds for the first time since my teen years.

Eventually I got as low as 186, and I found out something. I have pictures of the journey from the 199 to the 180s, but they are shirtless, and I know ain't nobody trying to see me posing shirtless and acting silly. Come to

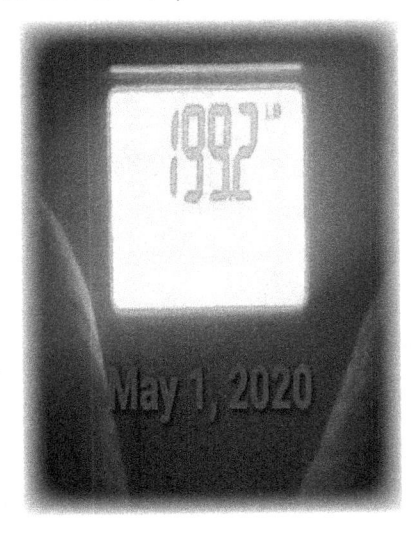

think of it, I wouldn't want to see it if I were you guys either.

I looked good, though. Take my word for it.

Interestingly enough, what I found was people may have hesitated to tell me I was too fat, but no one ever hesitated to tell me I was too skinny. They asked if I had cancer, AIDS, congestive heart failure, and some other diseases. A doctor from the hospital actually did a house call to my office to ask me if I was OK. My brother asked me if I was a crack-head—I *think* he was joking, but I'm still not sure.

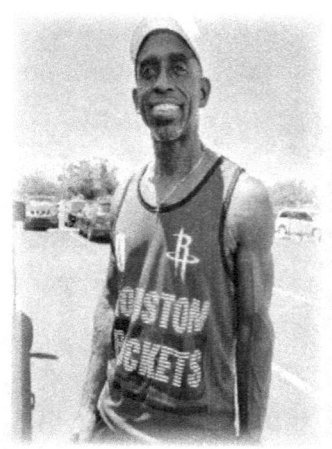

I was OK, but like I said, there was nothing to "stop." Still, though—I didn't want to weigh 186; it made me look older and sickly. I didn't want to weigh 320, either, because I love my feet. So I tinkered; I slowly reduced fasting and slowly added calories back in so I could stay in what I thought was my sweet spot—somewhere around 195.

I still count calories. Everything I've researched about intermittent fasting says there's no need to count calories, but I know that I must. It's like if I were a real playboy and trying to reform, I wouldn't go to the club; I wouldn't drink around dangerous women; I would be extra careful to avoid compromising situations. It's like gambling; a gamble-holic can go into the casino and drop $1,000 in thirty minutes, especially if they are the reckless type. It's the same thing for me and food; I'm a food playboy—an addict. And I tend toward recklessness; I can ingest two thousand calories or more in twenty minutes. I have to take precautions that normal people don't have to take.

I love my cheat days, though. I take one every twenty days just to relax my mind and control my playboy ways. I stay disciplined for those nineteen days because I know a Seafood Day is coming. I call them Seafood Days because on those days, I'll eat any food I see. I'll usually stop at around five thousand calories on Seafood Days, though. Usually.

Food playboy. For life.

I normally get back on my process the next day. Kind of. Don't judge me, nutritionists—I know binge eating is dangerously bad, and my readers know it too. Just trying to make a point.

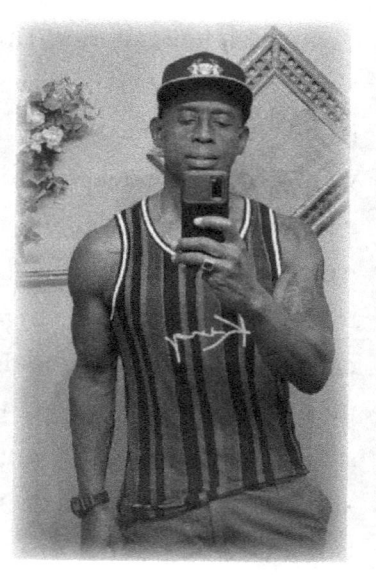

I exercise differently than I used to. I still get steps, but I get normal people steps, like ten thousand, or maybe twenty thousand if I'm feeling mega-froggy. I read that staying on the treadmill for an hour or running long distances increases estrogen and decreases testosterone. I found high-intensity interval training (HIIT) instead, which increases testosterone. Most people do HIIT by sprinting or doing something extra-vigorous for short periods, but my knees are bad. What I do is write one hundred body weight exercises on index cards—different kinds of jumping jacks, burpees, squats, planks, crunches, etc. Then I shuffle my cards and do whatever twenty cards come up first—ninety seconds of exercise, twenty seconds of rest. I started out doing thirty seconds of exercise and slowly increased over time.

And I don't exercise fast; I exercise slowly, as slow as I can possibly do the movement. I hold eight-, ten-, or fifteen-pound weights when I exercise whenever possible, and I don't count repetitions. There's no "do ten of these" or "do twenty of those." I do slow, controlled movements for ninety seconds, and however many I do…I do. Remember my cards? That's what I use. Told you I was a weirdo. I'm guessing there's an app or something that does this, but I'm old school, apparently. I trust my old, raggedy index cards.

Oh, and I love doing the Dumbbell Walk. Google "Farmers Walk," and you'll know what I'm talking about. I call it the Dumbbell Walk, though. Because I'm carrying dumbbells. Or because a dumbbell is walking. Take your pick. I thought it was clever.

I changed the way I fast too. Instead of counting my fasting hours daily, I count my fasting hours weekly. For example, I might declare a weekly goal of one hundred fasting hours; some days that week, I may want to fast twelve hours, some days twenty, some days I may not fast at all, but I try to hit that weekly goal. Women should fast that way, if they're going to do it. I'm no doctor, but a lot of research says women are more likely to get "hangry." It's because fasting reduces estrogen, the hormone women need. So women should start at seventy hours a week. Then go up two hours a week if and when they feel like it. Guys should start slow too. I'm no doctor; I already told you that. But that's what I did.

That's my story about going from about 320 or so down to 185, but I try to stay between 190 and 198 now. I'm not heavy anymore; I'm healthier than I have ever been. Some say when they look at my old pics that I look like my own grandson, which is kind of funny.

I remember when skinny people used to look crazy at me. I know they looked, and even if they never said it, we heavy people could feel their judgment, like they feel our size is disgusting, is our fault. They pity us or think we lack discipline. If you're skinny or in great shape and reading this right now, and you're a nice person, I'm not talking about you—thank you for buying my book.

But if you're skinny or in great shape and like to judge and criticize us like I described, cut it out… immediately.

And thank you for buying my book.

I'm sure I got judged, even though no one ever said anything to my face, but I'm focused on being nice to myself and not judging myself. Even now, I still don't chase pounds; I don't even chase appearance. There's a bunch of people who say I looked better when I was heavier.

Man, "the people" always got something to say, don't they?

But there were times I even looked at myself at 185 and thought, "Hey, what happened to my face?" It's clear to me that smaller is not always better.

So I stopped chasing pounds, and I stopped imagining I look better at this weight or that weight. I still chase the *clean*. I don't judge myself, and I reject others' judgment, too, at least as it pertains to my appearance.

I mean this as a compliment to myself: call me whatever you want, but I've got a fat-kid mentality, and I'm proud of it—which, for me, means you can judge my appearance however you want; I'm good with it. You can even say it out loud—I won't be up-set—but I'm more likely to be bothered if you tell me I'm dumb. Or uninteresting. Or mean.

You can congratulate me on losing weight, too, but the greater compliment is speaking to my intelli-gence, creativity, bravery, kindness, wisdom, or some other positive quality you see in me that doesn't go up and down like numbers on a weight scale. My fat-kid mentality means I see myself differently and reject *all* appearance judgments. Even my own. Be-cause I was a fat kid.

And mentally? I still am. And always will be.

I'm pretty proud of that.

AFTERWORD

IT'S MY TURN

THERE IS ABSOLUTELY *nothing* wrong with being considered "fat"—unless you're in the military, which will discharge you for not meeting their standards. But from a self-image standpoint, even in *that* case, there is nothing wrong with you if someone else believes you would be better off physically different from what you are right now. Like the same you, but with fewer pounds. Or with a different shape. Or with larger body parts. Or smaller body parts. Or softer parts. Or harder parts.

Listen, because I sincerely mean this: if you are healthy and happy with who you are, anyone—and I mean *anyone*—who is not likewise impressed should feel free to not look while you keep walking like a giant or giantess. Your size does not affect any of the combination of talents that makes you exciting, beautiful, uniquely special, and different from anyone else who has ever lived since the beginning of time. So go look in the mirror, and tell yourself that you're all that and then some (after you finish this last chapter). But if losing weight is what *you* want for yourself, you can do it; if I can do it, anybody can. Resilience is the key. When you try to boil it down to one word, it loses a lot of its power. It's not simply "bouncing back"; the details of resilience are the same principles we can all use to successfully navigate our journeys.

RESILIENCE IS PREPARATION

You can't just wait for challenging times to come, then hope you're ready for them; you must prepare in advance for the unknown. This weight loss journey also involves preparation; you can't wake up tomorrow and say, "Today's the day—time to drop a quick one hundred pounds." There are various methods, so do your research and pick one. I chose intermittent fasting and calorie counting; that worked for me, but something else may work better for you: keto, low fat, high fiber, Atkins, Weight Watchers, common-sense eating, and the list goes on. Exercise? I use high-intensity exercise, calisthenics, daily steps, and my beloved dumbbell walk, but you? Do you! Prepare, then pick something and plan to do it at the frequency that works for you. Do you know the most important thing that preparation involves? It's the mental aspect. Because no matter what method you pick, at some point, you will want to quit. At some point, you *will* quit. Probably because you're mad it's not working as fast as you want. Get ready for it, and decide in advance that when quitting day comes, the next day you're back on the grind. Don't call it a quitting day; call it a "rest day." And you rest so you can grind harder…so you can rest more…to grind harder. I think you understand this: you've got to get yourself ready. You've got to prepare.

RESILIENCE IS RECOVERY

Nobody wins all the time. Everyone loses eventually. It's one thing to plan for it, but it's a whole different thing when life socks you in the gut in an unexpected way and all you can internalize is, "Wow, that hurt. A lot. Way more than I thought it would." When life does that, the principle of resilience demands that you get up, because if you stay down, you lose. If you get up, you're back in the fight with a chance to win. I told you in the last section that you're going to have days where you did everything right and you still gained weight. Again. You're going to have days where you will be disappointed in your lack of [fill in the blank]. You're going to have days that start good but end with mouthfuls of chili cheese dogs and caramel cake that you know you shouldn't have, but you looked at something delicious and for that moment, you surrendered.

It's fine; it's even normal. (I just took a break from writing this paragraph to go eat too much banana bread—see?) It's OK, because you've prepared for it; you knew it was coming. When it happens, we're gonna get up. We're gonna shake it off. There's nothing to forgive, because we're human. No explanations, no excuses; we're gonna get up and get back to business. Fighters fight. I love saying that. Third time I've said it in this book, so it must be important.

RESILIENCE IS GROWTH

Life and the process of resilience demands that you learn from when you lose, so you get a little bit stronger, a little bit tougher, and a little bit smarter every time you fall, so hopefully, you can keep from creating or contributing to your own crises over and over and over again. As a matter of fact, life also demands that you learn and grow from your victories too, right? What'd you do? How did you do it? Can you do it again? And if you're anything like me, there have been times where you've won and you've thought, "Uhhh...I won? Wow, what a surprise!" Because sometimes I get lucky. Sometimes I win despite myself. Well, our journey mirrors life: we can learn when we lose, we can learn when we win, and we can learn when we get lucky. We have to remember our lessons; like for me, it was this:

Trust the process!

Fast longer!

Take breaks!

And no chili-cheese-dog-and-caramel-cake glutton-fests the day before I weigh in; I learned it the hard way.

Then you take all the lessons you learned, no matter what they were, and you make those lessons work for you. Use those lessons as you prepare some more. Because it's time to start the process all over again.

And in addition to those concepts of resilience, there are skills that science has shown will make you more resilient; I could cite the journal articles and studies, but I'm not trying to nerd out on you right now. Just don't use this book as the basis for any college papers or your thesis or anything, but take my word for it: these skills are legit. They will make you more resilient, and you can also apply them to your weight loss journey too. Like I did.

Physical resilience. We've talked about this already, but it's so important, I'll say it again: it's all mental. Forget the weight for a minute; your health and your longevity depend more than anything else on what you do and what you don't do. You get to choose, but remember, you can't cheat your body. You're going to pay what you owe. The same is true on your weight loss journey; you might lose a little, or you might lose a lot, but for the most part, it depends on what you do and don't do. So make good choices.

Capitalizing on strengths. Resilient people don't focus on what they don't do well and what doesn't work. They focus on their strengths; they identify the things they naturally do well; then they purposely use those strengths to make their lives stronger. Weight loss follows the same concept; I can't worry about what someone else does well or what they look like or anything that involves anyone else—it's all about me. And once I figured out I was a relentlessly meticulous individual who would weigh and write down everything he ate, I used it. I used my strengths to win, but first I had to find out what my strengths *were*.

Balance your thinking. Everyone has those moments in life where they thought later, "I wish I hadn't said that," "I wish I hadn't done that," or "I wish I hadn't thought that." Your weight loss journey will be filled with similar regrets; you know why? Unbalanced thinking! We have to stay out of those thinking traps, like "all or nothing." That's a trap—you're not going to lose the war because you had a bad day or two. Confirmation bias is also a trap: if you think you're going to lose, deep down, you will. The worst trap is blaming yourself; you've got to untie your self-image from the number on the scale. If your best friend called you right now and said, "I suck and I'm stupid and I'm ugly and I'm horrible because I didn't lose ten pounds this month," would you say, "Yes. I agree. You absolutely suck, loser. Just quit"?

No. You know what you'd tell your best friend in that situation—so tell yourself the same thing.

Optimism. When people fall, if they don't realize they can win, there's no reason to get up, is there? That happens in life all the time, so people have got to stay optimistic, just like everyone on a weight-loss journey. Because if you don't think you're going to win, why even go through all of this? Instead, trust the process, stay optimistic, ignore what appears to be a failure, and keep grinding no matter how long it takes. Not everyone will lose fifty, eighty, or one hundred pounds, and some of those who lose that much weight will gain it back. But you have to believe— you *have* to believe that you will meet your goal and you will maintain it. Keep thinking like a winner, and guess what happens? You win. Regardless of what number is on the scale or the size of your pants.

Purpose. This is your "why." Resilient people have developed a powerful, unseen driving force that compels them to keep going when life has dimmed the lights or completely turned them off. And it's that purpose that keeps them going, to keep fumbling around in the dark until they remember, "Wait, I know where that switch is!" Then they find it and switch the lights back on. That purpose can come from God, patriotism, race, gender, family name, profession, or from a set of qualities you've decided are how you will be defined.

For me, my weight loss journey was inspired by my feet. I didn't want to lose them. The doctor essentially said, "Want to keep your feet?" and my answer was "Yes, actually; I didn't know how much I loved my feet until you started talking about taking them away. They help me to walk. And I like walking way better than even pancakes." Purpose over pleasure, right? So find *your* purpose. And make it strong.

Mindfulness. The whole thing falls apart without this. Mindfulness is the ability to control where your mind goes and what it focuses on; resilient people don't let situations drive them or control their emotions. Instead of focusing on the inevitable hardships of life, resilient people stay focused on what their values are. Or what their strengths are. Or how they want to be viewed or what they want to be known for. Or their goals. Weight loss requires a similar focus because, as you know, it doesn't happen in a day or a week or a month. Then once you hit your mark, weight maintenance requires a similarly intense focus. Sometimes I take a mental break from it all and have a couple of pecan sticky buns. And some more stuff. But we can't focus on what we did wrong yesterday or last year. We've got to stay focused on the process. The skills and even your why won't matter as much if you forget it every time something happens you don't like.

And there you have it. Do I still wonder why no one ever told me I was fat? Nah…if they had, my feelings would have been hurt and…wait, someone *did* tell me, kind of. Mama and my Aunt Ann busted me in the kitchen one evening while I was on the hunt for buttered cornbread and syrup, as an *adult*, and gave me those side-eyed elder looks. You know the look I'm talking about, right? Then Mama rolled her eyes at Aunt Ann and said to me, "Are you hungry?" Then she said, all sarcastic, "Do you really need that extra piece of cornbread?" Yeah…in *that* voice.

"Let him eat, Rose. It's OK. I bet he *is* hungry."

That's my auntie. She's not the "Regulator Auntie"; she's the "always smiling, forever telling me how handsome I am, Vincent can do no wrong" kind of auntie.

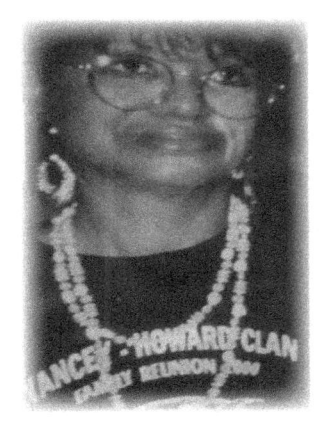

I think my auntie's words made me brave.

So I said, "No, ma'am—actually, I need *two pieces*!"

I thought I said it funny; my delivery was on point; I even made myself laugh—but I got smacked up anyway. Two smacks, really. None from my auntie. Mama got me twice with the double backhand. Mama and my aunt were both like that; they're from the "respect your elders" generation. They showed it differently, though. Aunt Ann was "Come dance with me"; Mama was "Get smart, and you get smacked." Different strokes, right?

I adore both of them—still had my two pieces of cornbread, though. And a third piece for good measure, just to show 'em who's boss. Drowned them in butter and syrup too.

It was pure coincidence that I waited to eat until they both went back in their rooms.

That's not specifically telling me I was fat, but it's close enough to show me that if anyone had told me

I was fat, that would have likely resulted in me eating even more. I hate being told what to do, which is a little odd for a thirty-year military guy, huh? Even if it results in a smack or two, I rebel a little bit when I get told what to do or get unsolicited advice. Sometimes I don't rebel a little; sometimes I rebel a lot.

Not being told I was fat may have worked in my favor. Instead of being told what to do and having a choice as to whether I would do the right thing, not being told allowed me to become *self-aware* and take responsibility for my own definition of the problem and my own fixes. And as any good coach knows, "I could tell you what to do and you might do it, but if you tell *yourself* what to do, then it's likely to stick."

And it has stuck. So far. But that's me. I misnamed this chapter, because the fact is that it's *your* turn now. If you're happy, stay happy. I'm still glad you bought the book, though, because you might decide you need a little inspiration for some journey in the future. If you're unhappy with your weight, health, or appearance, then let's get to work. I hope it's not appearance, though, because losing 120 pounds didn't make me any more handsome. Probably made me *less* handsome to some. More importantly, it didn't make me nicer or a better man or any smarter or kinder or anything like that; those things were always in me even when I was wearing XXL shirts and refusing to take pictures.

I promise you this, though. I'll never call you fat. I'm a "forever fat kid" mentally myself, but even if I did, who cares what I think? My opinion is irrelevant, and you know what? Nobody else should be calling you the *f*-word either or even thinking it, especially if you're kind, friendly, charismatic, talented, and soothing; everyone wants a friend like us.

But if you want to lose weight for *you*, that's OK too.

I did. I did it for my feet.

But I sure am glad nobody told me I was fat.

P.S.—My wife just told me while we were discussing this book to make sure that I put plenty of pictures in the book so that everyone would know that I really was very, very fat.

Her exact words.

Wow.

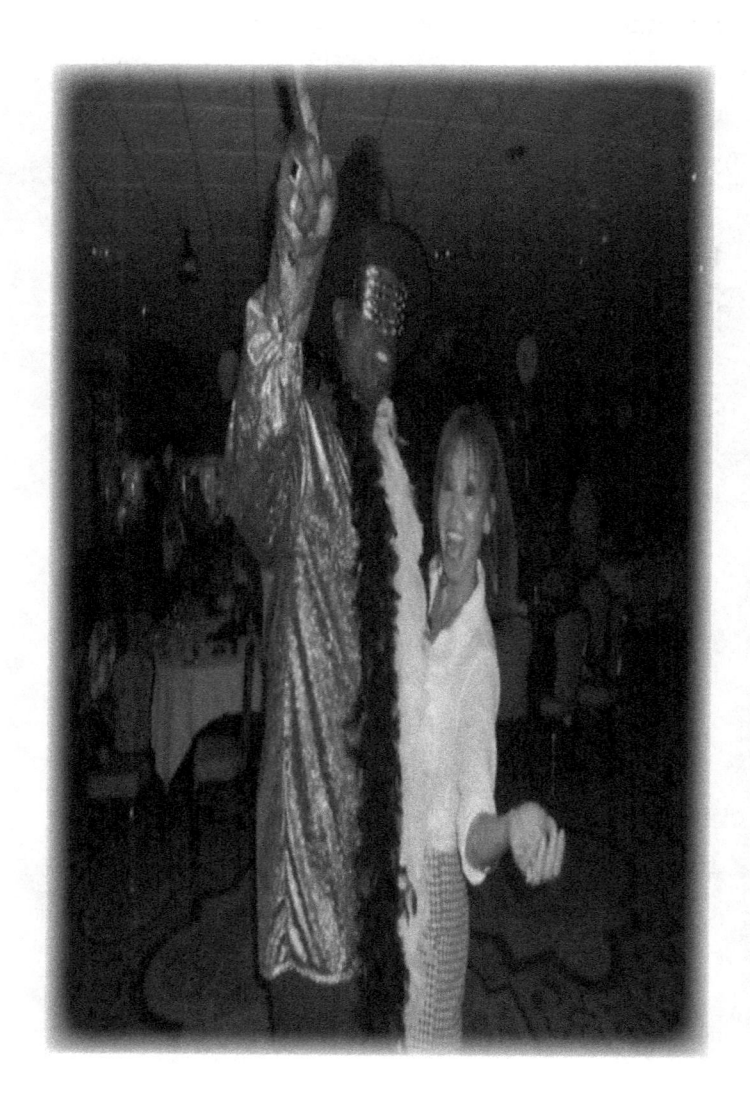

Printed in the USA
CPSIA information can be obtained
at www.ICGtesting.com
LVHW091241271023
762201LV00005B/901

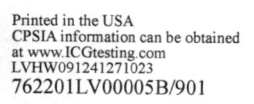

9 798822 920965